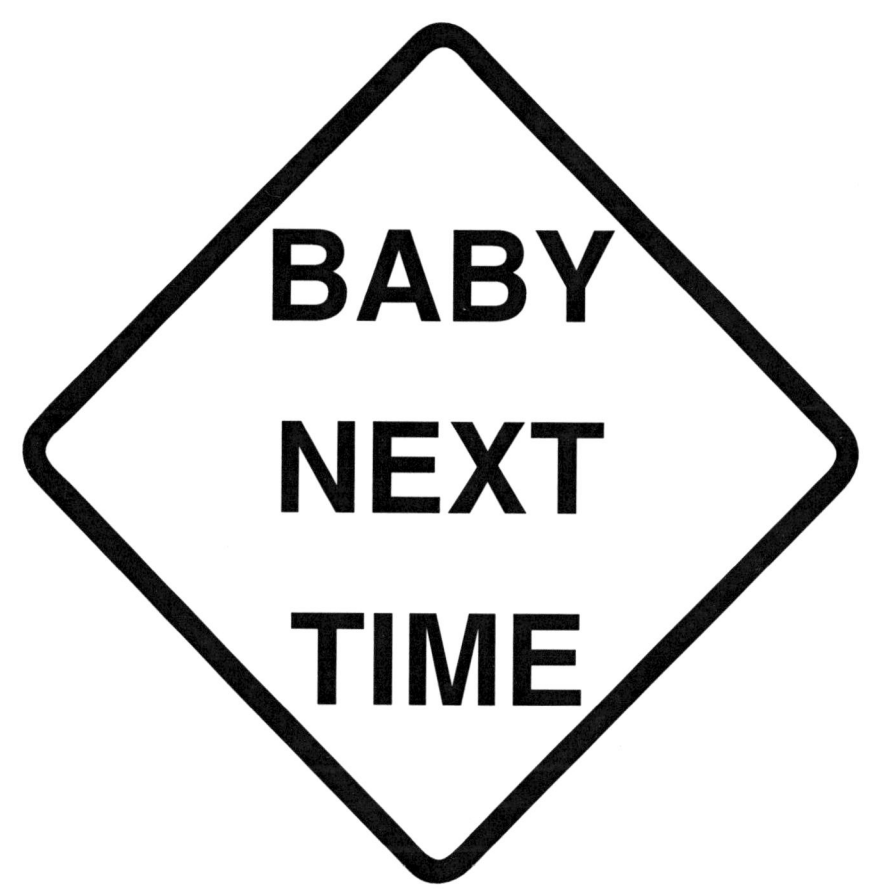

BABY NEXT TIME

by Nicole Klieff

AuthorHouse™
1663 Liberty Drive, Suite 200
Bloomington, IN 47403
www.authorhouse.com
Phone: 1-800-839-8640

First published by AuthorHouse   1/29/2009

ISBN: 978-1-4343-9512-2 (sc)
ISBN: 978-1-4343-9513-9 (hc)

Printed in the United States of America
Bloomington, Indiana

This book is printed on acid-free paper.

authorHOUSE®

To Gerry and Peter
Your memory will live on

Chapter One

*M*y earliest memories as a child regarding babies was the etched out pain from watching women giving birth in television dramas, thinking there was no way on earth I was going to put myself through that! Another very early memory was putting myself into a semi-trance and thinking that if I sat on a public toilet for too long some little green men would suck me down the loo and flush me out pregnant.

As I matured, having been taught the facts of life, I wandered into the world of dating and comparing notes with friends over sexual exploits and the best contraception methods to use. Getting married and having babies was far away on the agenda.

During my 20s I enjoyed and became more involved with the prospects of a demanding career. I was working within the record industry. I worked in the centre of town. It was all happening. This was the path to follow. It was the 1980s. Maggie Thatcher was in government. Ladies now had growing ambitions. Make money, have an apartment, travel and just lap up the opportunities for total independence.

I just assumed that when I met the right guy everything else would fall into place.

Like any other young girl it was preached that little girls change shape, expect a monthly bleed, marry, have children and eventually enjoy being a grandmother.

Some twenty years later nothing prepared me for the anxieties of not being able to conceive or the disappointments of having miscarriages. Doctors consistently telling me and my husband that "we were categorised under the definition of inexplicable reasons as to why you both are not able to have a full-term pregnancy".

This world at first was very foreign but eventually it was to become my world; and as the expression goes, "welcome to the real world". Nothing could have prepared me for the experience of the roller-coaster ride of undergoing fertility treatments in our quest to have a baby. Certainly at the offset if you had told me I would experience this over a nine-year period I would never have believed it and would have replied "that would be absolute obsessive madness". Indeed this did happen but not out of choice and not always with treatment.

Let me start from the beginning of our journey to have a baby. I met my husband in 1992 after being engaged to marry a complete jerk who incidentally had been engaged six times previous but that is another story.

This original wedding was to have taken place in June 1992. It was to be on a grand scale and my father had saved for many years for the day to arrive when he would give away his only daughter. To this day it still breaks my heart that I had to tell him the wedding was off. My fiancé didn't even have the balls to face him. The engagement broke up just eight weeks prior to the actual wedding date in June. It was over a long Easter weekend in April. I was

32 years old, broken-hearted and most of all angry. Looking back now it was also a relief as I certainly had a lucky escape. The whole liaison was wrong. However, I was disappointed and felt isolated at the time.

One by one my friends were edging away, fulfilling their own journeys of life. Slow death of detachment. Of course they had their own lives to live and were now at "marital age" and babies were being born left, right and centre. The basic denominator was not there for me. I lost contact with many, as now I did not fit into their world.

I decided that something had to change. I could be faced with being left on the shelf and certainly did not want to be a bitter old woman with nothing to show. This was just not me. At the same time I would rather be single, happy and free with choices rather than in a trapped, mundane and loveless marriage, just being a baby producing machine.

So a career change was on the horizon and I jumped at the opportunity. I decided to enter the world of sales, facing the pressures of meeting targets - making as much money as I could. Indeed this took up plenty of my time and I was quite happy to retreat back to my studio apartment, indulging in TV dinners, keeping up to date with the soaps, speaking hours on the telephone to the few close social friends I had left. Mobile phones were then not in full operation.

It was on a balmy evening back in June 1992 that the phone rang and a platonic male friend invited me to join him and a few friends for a bite to eat at a new Pizza restaurant in Belsize Park. I remember it like yesterday as it was probably one of the first times I ventured out socialising after the broken engagement. It was one very strange, fun and different evening and little did I know at the time, this was the evening I would meet my husband to be.

We were a party of five but I was the only female there as another dropped out at the last minute. I knew none of the other three people invited. My host and I arrived first and then in walked this very tall, broad, dark-haired larger than life handsome man. His profession - a magician. He proudly told me that he belonged to the magic circle and was travelling within the United States, appearing on television networks doing his tricks. His name was Alan.

Then the two other invited guests, both men, walked into the restaurant and introduced themselves. One of the men, Barry, was very short, skinny, badly dressed but with a pleasant, easy-go-lucky manner, and the other, Michael, was very tall, spotty and extremely shy.

Alan took over the table and indeed the restaurant. He did his tricks and entertained us and in fact attracted onlookers from other tables. He was also very flirtatious and didn't waste time on asking me out on a date.

A few days later I received a phone call from Barry who also asked if I would go on a date with him. I agreed and we spent a lovely evening together and it was on this date that he announced that we would marry and that he would like to be the father of my children!

I retreated after that date. I had undergone a broken engagement and the last thing I wanted to do was start a serious relationship at that point, leading to engagement of marriage and getting pregnant. I was not ready. Instead a holiday was more appealing and so I took myself off. On my return I had received messages from both Alan and Barry saying that they wanted to get together again.

On the evening of going out with Alan, he cancelled and was never to be seen again. I stayed at home. Later that same evening I received a call from Barry and we arranged a date for the following evening.

We met up and, to my surprise after the previous meeting, I really enjoyed being in his company and we just clicked. We dated for another six months, fell in love and then started to live together. We co-habited for a year before Barry proposed marriage. Everything was healthy and blissfully happy. My life now was taking shape. We were planning the future and saving to move from the flat we shared to enable us to purchase a house to bring up a family.

In June 1994 we had a wonderful wedding arranged by my parents who, despite the disappointment of the previous cancelled wedding, did a brilliant job. We were surrounded by family and close friends and had never been happier. Nothing too ostentatious but a wedding that suited both our personalities. We honeymooned in Sardinia and took an extra week off at the flat. We eventually returned back to work striving for the new house which we found and moved into 18 months later.

It was also at this time that I decided to leave the hospitality agency where I'd been working and set up on my own. This was feasible as the type of work required just a phone and computer, and the names of all my contacts and clients.

I had worked at a well-known corporate hospitality agency based at Wembley Stadium for four years. I had four years' sales experience. I was selling hospitality packages to all businesses, to entertain their clients at major sporting and music events.

There were sales targets that had to be met and I was also involved in cold calling to key decision makers.

In order to lessen the stress and to be able to have a baby, I decided that it was a good time to leave in view of the imminent changes that were happening within Wembley at that time. As staff we were shunted from pillar to post from one office to another because of the impending building works. I was also fed up with the 'whip and do' method and wanted to work at my own pace.

When I did set up I was amazed and grateful for the many clients that did follow me and have happily continued helping them with their requests to this day. Without their help I probably would not have been able to financially contribute to the forthcoming fertility treatment we required.

I also had a client who, as a chemist, offered to help me find cheaper drugs for IVF treatment, should I require them.

I must admit it was great working from home even though the pennies were much harder to earn. No commuting, no whip, not witnessing the next announcement of a new baby on the horizon and no bitching. I was relaxed and more comfortable, and focused on what was a new and happy experience.

It was during the following year that we decided that Barry and I would take the next step - HAVING A BABY. Arrogantly we thought it would be easy and we would be holding our bundle of joy after our move to the new house.

We both had check-ups at the local medical centre. Our GP told us we were both in good health and despite the fact that I had passed the so called peak (I was then aged 35) in a woman's cycle, should have no trouble conceiving and wished us luck. We enthusiastically started our mission.

For the first six months we chose to ignore the fact that my periods rolled again and again. We told ourselves that it would happen sooner or later and continued in our bid to become parents.

After 18 months of frustration, the situation was starting to change. I was becoming moody and short tempered. I began to lose focus on topping sales at work. I seemed to be frequently on the verge of tears, especially if I was out shopping and saw a pregnant woman or one of the endless numbers of strollers and prams with a cute baby or toddler on board. This also extended to holding back anxieties when speaking to friends who were already experiencing the trials and tribulations of parenthood. Both Barry and I found it extremely difficult to become acquainted with new friends too. Being the age we were it seemed everyone we met was either pregnant or talking about their child's first tooth, new shoes, or what school to attend. It was also difficult to arrange meeting friends in the evening as many would use the excuse, no babysitter this week, let's make a date in the unforeseeable future.

We would often question if these excuses were plausible as we became conscious of the fact that people began to feel uncomfortable in our presence because we were a childless couple. I must admit this applied even more once we undertook treatment later down the line, and indeed we became more reclusive.

So why could I not be a mummy? What was I doing wrong? How come all these other women could do it and I couldn't? What was wrong with me?

I started to feel guilty for leaving it so late. However, it seemed that destiny had stepped in. The opportunity of meeting the right partner had only recently occurred. I felt guilty for not looking after my fitness level - maybe I should have gone back to playing squash, started swimming again and cut down on the smoking but there again I did not drink alcohol. No one is perfect. I also questioned whether it was maybe time to leave my job? Get away from the pressures of trying to reach company sales targets and rushing about meeting deadlines. Avoid stressful situations. Easier said than done, as one has to earn a living.

I started to question Barry; what if he was "shooting blanks"? Would he be prepared to find out and get tested? The same applied to me. Why could I not produce healthy eggs? I had always felt strong and healthy, so much so that I boasted to people that I never got colds or flu. I am not a sickly person. The occasional zit, the odd backache, rheumatic pains, yes indeed, but probably due to lack of physical exercise. I had, in fact, been prone to rheumatic pains even during my teenage years, which I partially blamed on the fact that I participated in championship swimming and during later years participated only in swimming on my twice yearly holiday travels. (At a later stage it became apparent that this was a problem.) At work and play I had become a bum-on-seat person. I began to change certain parts of my diet to fit in with the trends of the time, many of which had been reported as helping with fertility.

I was literally questioning everything to the point of becoming obsessed. We even took the moon into account as I had discovered something called the 'biorhythmic lunar cycle', in which research seemed to show that a woman is at her most fertile during her lunar peak, i.e. at the same phase of the moon that was present at birth. Full moons were certainly nights where we would use all our endeavours to pursue pregnancy. We even followed the standard horoscope readings to ascertain whether our luck would be in! Both Barry and I have the same star-sign. We are sensitive cancerians.

Eventually we got all these feelings of resentment and fears out in the open. We had a long heart to heart talk and agreed that, as an equal team and with our love for each other, standing side by side, we could get through this together, and decided we needed to get some answers from the professionals.

We paid a visit to the GP who referred us to an obstetrician based in Harley Street. Little did we know at the time that this was only the beginning of what would be a long physical, expensive and emotional journey and above all a true test on the survival of our marriage.

Chapter Two

When we first went to see an obstetrician (OB) we had been referred from our GP; we told him how exasperated we were in our bid to have a baby.

The OB was based in Harley Street and with plenty of years experience on this subject. He gave us the impression that our choice to have a baby should not be too much of a problem.

We had preliminary tests together and I was prescribed Clomid tablets. They were supposed to enhance the quality of ovulation. It is an anti-estrogen which tricks the pituitary gland into producing the hormones that stimulate ovaries. The course I had was a gradual build-up, starting with the minimum and ending up with maximum dosage over several months, which seemed an eternity.

Whilst on this course I also took temperature readings from a specialised thermometer. A certain temperature reading would inform us if ovulation was indeed happening.

This was followed by progesterone injections used to thicken the lining of the uterus. These were administered to assist ovulation.

Then a blood test would follow. My arms were like an old has-been dart board from all the blood tests and my hips were swollen from the intramuscular injections. I was red, black and blue!

It became a weekly task of travelling to and fro through London's busy streets in between work.

I have a very vivid memory when, after a visit to the laboratories based in Harley Street on a bright sunny day, I was walking down Marylebone High Street on my return to work. I was wearing a gleaming white long-sleeved blouse which wasn't too revealing; however, I became conscious of the constant stares of passers by. I took a glance at what I was wearing and was totally aghast to discover that one arm was saturated in blood, and I mean saturated. People must have been wondering who I'd murdered - was it a person or a spaniel? What do you do? I rushed back to the pathology (blood-test) laboratories and the nurses who attended to me just laughed it off. "The cotton wool ball and bandage fell off. It happens from time to time - we'll clean it up. You are just one big bleeder." Take it from me, it's not what you want to hear and see.

To top it all, when I returned to my car a glistening parking ticket had been stamped across my window screen. I felt physically sick and angry.

I was angry, not so much because of the blood incident, but rather because of the parking fine. We were already paying money on a regular basis for me to have the drugs during ovulation. This was accompanied by the weekly blood tests to analyse the situation. Having said that, due to the fact we were still at the investigative stage, medical insurance was acceptable but the initial outlay had to come from us before we were reimbursed, slowly.

I remember an incident when I had to renew my insurance policy explaining that I came under investigatory on reasons why

I couldn't fall pregnant and that the treatment involved would include many exploratory tests on a regular basis. I also asked the question "would this cover IVF treatment". The telephone adviser was unsure and he replied insensitively "well most people do not need IVF, you are not the norm". Ouch!

The reason that we had to take up a private medical scheme in the first place was because once you are over the age of 35, in this country, no fertility treatment is given on the NHS unless, as I believe, you live within a certain postcode area and even then the goalposts are moved over and over again each year.

Another memory was when my ovulation cycle fell on a weekend and at that stage I needed someone to administer the injection that was required. I hated injections/needles and can't watch the needle pierce into skin even to this day. Thankfully my OB's lovely assistant invited me to her flat in North London and did the deed, for which I was truly grateful and relieved that I did not have to administer the needle myself; little did I know at the time that that would all change later, big time!

It was a very trying time, sitting in traffic facing the latest 'baby on board' sign, travelling back and forth through London to be pierced by a needle, sitting in waiting rooms, which of course included seeing very pregnant women, collecting bruises, losing money and ensuring that I would be relaxed enough when home to connect with the right temperature reading and catch a swimming sperm having swallowed the Clomid pills.

Side effects were another issue I was uncomfortable with but was assured that nothing too untoward would happen. I took Clomid for around a year and after abandoning it, I remember turning on the car radio and hearing that after prolonged use, this could be associated with an increased risk for ovarian cancer. Apparently they are still researching this! The desire to have a child was even stronger by then and it was too late to query the dangers.

After a good year or so of this course of medication 'it weren't working' - changes were needed.

My OB suggested that I have an operation called a Laparoscopy. This allows the physicians to see the outside of the uterus, ovaries and fallopian tubes. In short, everything internal. I would be put under anaesthetic and a small camera would be inserted through the belly-button area in order to have a peek.

I was booked into a hospital off Harley Street. The admission date was 6 May 1999 (I was fast approaching the age of 39). I was to be a day-patient and to check-in at 7.00 a.m. I was very apprehensive at the time as I had never been under anaesthetic during my adult life and this was to be a first-time experience but once again the drive to have a child took over.

I woke up to what felt like a period. Achy, a little blood flow and I remember backache as if I had been kicked by a whole football team. I was told later that it was from the carbon dioxide to inflate the abdomen and was given painkillers to aid the pain.

When Barry and I got home that evening I ate for every baby born that day! I couldn't have anything at home the night before and the hospital food during the day was what we all expect of hospital food. It was easy to fill the bloated tummy and oh how I wished if only a baby could fill it instead.

The results showed that nothing was out of place; yes one of my ovaries was slightly smaller than the other but then so are feet! I certainly should not have any problem producing eggs. I was reassured that this was not the problem.

Our OB suggested that he would refer us to go for the 'full Monty' by having fertility treatment at a well-known fertility clinic or continue with his methods. He backed it up with the view that because we came under 'inexplicable' it might be an emotional and difficult time with no guarantees of a result at the end.

We were thoroughly disillusioned and despondent at not having discovered the reasons for our 'inexplicable' infertility and we went home, had a discussion and did our sums. We agreed that we now had no option but to go to the recommended fertility clinic and to see what the next move would entail.

My OB wrote his referral letter and at the end of June 1999, a couple of days after my 39th birthday, we were invited to an open evening. The clinic is located in central London not far from a bridge. After parking nearby and taking what was to become a regular walk over the bridge, on that summer's evening Barry and I literally held our breath with anticipation.

When we arrived we were offered refreshments and started chatting with some of the attendees. It was a very relaxed atmosphere for a serious confrontation. During the seminar we were given an introduction about the different procedures/facilities/treatments available/percentage charts showing success/failure rates. We were given a tour of the different rooms.

I looked around at the other attendees. People were from all nationalities and backgrounds. Some even attended with children in tow.

A woman who sat next to me revealed she was in her late forties and this was her final chance. I thought she was very brave but it was unusual. Was I in a position to judge? As I discovered, age discrimination can be mixed with naivety. Sometimes allowances have to be made and individually assessed. We are all made differently and sometimes the results from life are too. We have to take what is dealt and deal with it the best way we can in order to follow our destiny. Ageism can be a bitch!

The person giving the seminar was the clinic director, an attractive man. Personally, he reminded me of a younger version of Omar Sharif, the actor. He was running the shop and it was a very expensive one!

Chapter Three

After having signed all the entry and permission forms for treatment to take place, an appointment had been made for us to be assessed by the clinic's director himself.

A mid-afternoon appointment on Wednesday 14 July had been arranged, exactly a week after Barry's 42nd birthday. I remember it being the afternoon as we were still at the clinic late in the day and it was not so crowded and busy.

We arrived to check into the reception to then be directed to a very crowded waiting room. This was a very depressing room. The atmosphere was heavy with sadness. Every seat was taken. Barry and I eventually were able to sit to face the onslaught of unhappy faces. I noticed that some people were clutching onto heavy files of paper for dear life, holding specimen pots and you could feel the butterflies of nerves that day! So much so, the coffee machine in the corner was on over-time and ran out of water not just on that day but several times on each of my visits.

Occasionally the television, which was perched high up on the wall with a slightly blurred picture, would be the only sound heard, blurting out with the latest depressing news, or day time magazine programmes concentrating on problems and dilemmas, or churlish daytime soaps to reel people's minds from the task in hand. I personally found it irritating.

The magazines left out were not much better to read. The choice was poor and being always out-of-date and generally teeny! The other alternative was to read the pamphlets on how to become pregnant or why you are not getting pregnant. What to do with baby if you were lucky enough to have one.

My experience of waiting in this room was to just sit quietly and sip at water from the triangular cups as given from the water stand in the opposite corner to the frequently used coffee machine and to think of England - anything other than what was to come. I knew, however, that this would not be my last visit to this room. Bottom line, like everyone else in that room, I did not want to be there but I had no choice if I wanted to have a baby.

Prior to meeting the fertility director, we were subjected to take on yet more tests. It had been arranged that I was to have an ultrasound scan with blood tests. Barry was also required to have blood tests and to participate in yet another sperm test. We were ushered to what I can only describe as a box room. No windows, no natural light, just a couple of chairs, a bed and boxes of medical appliances, i.e. syringes, bandages, and syringe disposal units. We both had our blood taken by a very nice bouncy smiley nurse. Barry and I were then separated in order for me to have the ultrasound and Barry to have his semen tested.

His experience was described to me in graphic terms, explaining to how difficult it is to produce a sperm sample. He went into a small room, with no window. There was a toilet, wash-hand basin and a small two-seater sofa. On it were a stack of well thumb girlie magazines.

He was provided with a small plastic container. The trick was to ejaculate into the cup which was not quite as easy as he first thought. He had to cover his penis with the cup; therefore the cup was upside down at this point, defeating the object of the exercise. He said he had to hold back and manoeuvre his penis in order to catch the semen into the container without any spillage. After he had done the deed, he got dressed, washed and left the room which led into a small lobby area where there was a hatch. He rang the bell at the side of the hatch and waited. A woman on the other side opened the hatch door and with a latex gloved hand took the sample, never to be seen again! Barry was informed that his sperm count was normal. So did the problem lay with me?

I was taken to a larger room whereby there was an open hatch within the wall and TV screen attached to the wall above. The main attraction was a rectangular table (bed) plonked in the centre of the room with imposing stirrups attached at the end. The bed was covered with a sheet of flimsy paper. This was a scary sight; memories came flooding back to those early childhood nightmares from the movies! To the right of the bed was a host of scanning equipment.

I was told to strip waist down and to plaster myself on to this monstrosity of a bed. I was to lie on top of the bed and then instructed that my backside had to be sat towards the end of the bed. Unfortunately this proved to be a difficult task as the paper which was placed on the top of the bed constantly slipped off and move me with it. Nervous giggles filled the room.

Eventually I was successfully perched towards the end of the bed with my backside finally attached to the paper sheet beneath me. I was instructed that my legs were to be raised in the air spread apart with feet laid through each of the stirrups. I remember the nurse putting on the jelly-like substance across my stomach and me responding with a winced face and a yelp "bloody hell, that's freezing!" Never mind the groping going on with the inspection of my internal organs/private parts at the other end of the bed.

The reason for the jelly was so that an object similar to a computer mouse would be scrolled over my stomach so that it was easier to view the internal organs and investigate the state of the ovaries and the lining of the uterus. I took a sneaky look at the screen to see if I could recognise anything. I didn't. All I saw was a huge black hole within my tummy. It was pointed out that everything was in good order - no cysts could be felt or seen. Fallopian tubes clear, as were ovaries. The lining of the uterus was as it should be at that time of the month.

I was then told to get dressed and return to the original little box room. Barry returned to the room shortly after. Whilst the nurse was not in the room we quickly exchanged notes of what had just gone on before being interrupted mid-way by the return of the happy go-lucky smiley face. She was about one of the only people there that smiled. She was always a pleasure to see. Good mood or not! She ushered us back to the original waiting room to be greeted by fewer glum faces.

It seemed an eternity as we were kept waiting. One by one the room was emptying until eventually we were the only people left. It was a good job that we had taken the whole afternoon off work!

Eventually we were greeted by the fertility director. As we walked down the corridors the walls were plastered with baby pictures - success stories no doubt!

The meeting with the fertility director was basically a lesson on why things possibly were not working. He reviewed our previous course of treatment, including the laparoscopy which I had undergone. He drew diagrams of my internal organs outlining what possibly could be the problem, and finally explained the treatment we were to undergo. He also pointed out that 25-30% of cases would fail, for unexplained reasons, to fall pregnant.

He went on to say that as both Barry and I showed no signs of problems (OK, right, then how come it had already taken four years with nothing to show?), that he recommended we should undergo artificial insemination, Intra Uterine Insemination, also known as IUI.

Before we left we filled out and signed more forms and were also given a prescription to collect from the clinic's pharmacy for the drugs to be used for this course of treatment.

Another reason for going down this route at the time was because we were told it was financially a better option. The drugs alone cost close to £1,500. The cost to have this procedure (IUI) was considerably cheaper, at about £1,000, as opposed to full-blown IVF, which would cost over £2,000 without the drugs. To this day we still have the original bills. Maybe subconsciously we thought we could have a refund if it did not work.

Believe me, we scrimped and scraped a huge amount of savings that we had put aside, missing out on many treats we had previously planned. It was a gamble but we both decided we had no other option; we wanted our child, our heritage to continue. Unfair as it seemed, if we had to pay so be it. We were on our own. We were too old to go via the NHS route; however, it was at the time discretionary for your local GP to prescribe the drugs. No medical insurance policy would cover IVF treatment.

IUI is similar to the full blown version of IVF in its usage of fertility drugs, blood tests and scans to ascertain if and when ovulation was occurring. The difference, however, was that when ovulation did take place in this instance, I would experience no more than the recent ejaculated sperm mixed with my eggs being injected into my womb by a catheter. The date was 6 September 1999. I remember it being a very quick and painless procedure.

The IUI procedure was certainly more direct and less complicated than what we might have to endure further down the road if we were to be unsuccessful, although the inception of the drugs on a daily basis was unforgiving.

After the insertion, I was instructed to take things easier, avoid stressful situations but to continue life as normal, whatever that means. I was to return in two weeks time after carrying out a pregnancy test. This wait was the longest two weeks you can endure during fertility treatment. The discipline in trying to stay cool and collected is difficult. Life goes on!

We returned to work and continued with our regular chores as if nothing was going on but quietly holding our breath, literally! It was a nervy time for both of us and anyone else who has been down this road will tell you the same.

Possibly it was harder for me because as well as dealing with the day to day situations, my hormones were all over the place! My body felt ugly, being very bloated and bruised and I just generally felt very tender with every move. Hot flushes, and feeling tired were also symptoms. I had a constant metallic taste in my mouth which was the feedback from taking the drugs. The mood swings and anguish I endured also added to feeling lousy.

I woke up two weeks later to a beautiful clear blue sunny morning. Barry and I were like two nervous teenagers about to embark on the unknown. My period had not turned up. For the past week whenever I went to the loo, I would take a quick glance to see if any blood had deposited itself on my knickers.

This morning was the day we had waited for with baited breath. It was the day to pee on the famous dipstick known as a pregnancy test. I went to the bathroom and closed the door behind me shaking with the anticipation. There is a transparent window indented on the stick. If a blue line appeared within the window, I was pregnant. If not, then it was back to the drawing board. I waited a minute or two as instructed; nothing altered. I took a second test as I did not want to believe it. No change. I fought back the tears and came out of the bathroom to be greeted by the biggest hug and cuddle. Barry knew just by looking at me the result!

On reflection, looking back, we should never have gone ahead with this procedure and should have taken the route of full-blown IVF to have maximised our chances. You follow the experts, 'the doctors know best' routine. Both Barry and I naively didn't question whether it would be right for us. You don't, do you, when you see experts?

After getting rid of the two pregnancy test sticks, Barry and I took the day off work and had a late leisured breakfast and talked and talked till we could talk no more. We discovered that deep down both of us thought this might not work and were now eager to go through the next stage as we thought surely our chances would be better. We also knew we would have to be put on a waiting list so we had to act quickly. The clock was ticking fast!

I rang the clinic informing them of the result and they expressed their sorrow. An appointment was arranged for a check over and to discuss what was to be the next move.

The following day to my disappointment my period arrived. It was the full confirmation before going to the clinic.

Chapter Four

We arrived at the reception of the clinic to be greeted by the familiar smiley nurse who was chatting with the receptionist. It was as if she was waiting for us. She offered her sadness on our failure to succeed in our endeavours. We were told to go to the waiting room to wait our turn before being ushered to see the fertility director. Hated that room!

Once again we were kept waiting due to the fact that he was in surgery. Generally speaking it was explained that theatre would take place in the morning and that as soon as he had done his business he would come out and speak to us.

The wait was not as bad as we first thought. About 20 minutes later, he appeared in his blue overalls with his clipboard holding our written updates and ushered us into his office. He was sorry that we had not be successful and immediately encouraged us to proceed with IVF treatment as soon as possible in order to maximise our chances. This, as he explained, was due to the fact that the continuation of using the fertility drugs added to what I had already utilised could be of benefit in optimising our success. He also indicated that the drug intake would increase but the application would be similar to what I had already undergone.

He wrote out a prescription similar to what we had previously received, the only difference was that he had increased the dosage of Gonal-F (used for stimulation of follicular growth and ovulation - given by subcutaneous injections) by more units. I was prescribed a higher level of a down regulation drug called Synarel (nafarelin) also known as a LH-RH analogue. This suppresses the production of hormones which stimulates the ovaries to develop follicles. After using this for a fortnight, the normal function of my ovaries would be switched off. It allows for greater control over the development of the follicles in response to the Gonal F and prevents spontaneous ovulation.

I would have to sniff the Synarel, a nasal spray, through my nostrils three times a day.

In simple language I will try to explain what this meant but as you can appreciate, like probably most of you reading this account, I am not a medical expert but will try to express it in a language easier to understand.

Barry indicated that since he had to give the injections, he wanted reassurance that he was doing so correctly. The nurse demonstrated how to administer the subcutaneous and intramuscular injections that would be required. We were also given the needles and syringes, together with the disposal waste box for getting rid of the used needles. The nurse wished us the best of British, before we collected our prescription, which had been left at the reception desk on the route out!

Prior to leaving the building we had to pay our deposit for the forthcoming treatment. We also planned to visit our GP to see if perhaps he could supply us with the recommended drugs.

To our relief and joy, our GP got the permission to write out the prescription. A visit to chemist was the next place of call.

During the IUI treatment I went back and forwards to the clinic in order to receive the fertility injections from a nurse on a daily basis, as well as having ultrasound appointments to follow progress. Driving through the London traffic proved to be an added stress I could have well done without.

The other alternative was to go to my local GP but I did not fancy sitting in a waiting room full of germs for hours on end on a daily basis.

Like clockwork my period started on time the following month (October) and I started to sniff the nasal spray.

On the fifth day of my cycle I would go to the clinic for an ultrasound. I would then be told when I could commence the fertility injections (Gonal-F). If I was not ready, I would return in a couple days for another scan before the go-ahead. I was also a walking bathroom cabinet. I rattled so much from all the pills I was swallowing!

Barry would then administer the injections on a nightly basis as instructed by the nurse. He became a proper little nurse! In short he would have to inject on my backside or fatty hips. It was not Barry's fault I was becoming sorer and bruised as the nightly routine continued; it was all part of the process.

After a week or so I would be expected to go to the clinic for a scan to assess the number and size of the developing follicles. These scans would apply a couple of times more if the follicles had not reached the appropriate size. Often I would have some follicles that had, and then have to wait in hope that the others would catch up. Having said that, I was told that the number of follicles shown on the ultrasound did not guarantee the number of eggs collected as some of the follicles were empty.

When you are ready for your egg collection, the hCG injection (Profasi) is administered if the ultrasound shows that there has been growth on the follicular development from the daily usage of Gonal F. The Profasi injection is to help mature the eggs within the follicles. In short, this injection will trigger ovulation.

Barry and I called this "the big one", as this was the last one given around midnight, approximately 36 hours before the operation. You could only administer this if you were ready for egg collection as confirmed by the ultrasound hours earlier. It was also at this time that I was instructed to finish using the nasal spray.

It was 7.30 in the morning on 4 November 1999, the day before Guy Fawkes. Our fireworks were starting a day earlier. It was IVF day!

In the main reception of the hospital there was an open lounge. We were told to report here to check in. There were three other couples looking just as bleary-eyed. An observation I made at the time was that beside each of the women there was an overnight bag. The funny side to this was that we were all only to be there for a day. We would be provided with a gown and could not wear any make-up or nail-polish. We could not eat or drink. Not even a glass of water, which I was dying for! I laughed to myself - we are creatures of habit!

After signing the admission form for the operation, we were directed to our room. I was terrified! Never mind blood in my knickers I was crapping myself.

Once in my room, Barry and I kissed each other bye byes, and he was ushered away to do yet another semen specimen. He was told that there was no point him being at the clinic as I would be unconscious for quite sometime and be groggy until the middle of the afternoon.

I changed into the hospital gown which was laid on the bed neatly pressed and folded. A nurse took my blood pressure, pulse and weight before a doctor who I had never met before came in. She explained the procedure and asked me if I had any questions and was I OK. Underneath I was neurotic but I replied that everything was cool!

The operation was to be performed under general anaesthetic and I remember being wheeled towards a large lift. We were then going down. The doors opened to a typical hospital corridor, with the smell of antiseptic bouncing off the walls. I was being wheeled to my final destination which was a stark cold clinical room with ample florescent lighting! I remember staring up to a few people standing around my movable bed assessing what hand had the best veins. Each of them introducing themselves individually and being generally chatty. My thoughts were get it over and done with, please. Ouch! Unconscious!

When I woke up I heard muffled voices around me. Directly in front of me I saw a pair of vertical bare feet. I was groggy and no way on earth could I lift up my head. I moved my eyes to the left of me where a nurse was assisting a nearby patient. I then glanced to my right and saw a lady bowing her head over the side of her bed to sip water from a plastic cup. I was in foreign land!

I closed my eyes for another minute or two before a female voice asked "would you like a drink of water?" I took the paper cup and she assisted me in my endeavours to drink. She then vanished and I lay staring at the ceiling another five minutes or so before she came back to discover I was more alert to respond to her. She was excitedly telling me that they had managed to collect nine. Some were at a good size. At first I thought she meant eggs and as I came to, I realised she was talking about follicles. I responded by saying "that's great!" I did not have a clue what the average was. She told me that that was the above average rate. This was really a numbers game, a true lottery in every sense of the word!

Shortly after the attendees returned me back to my bed and a nurse came in to the room offering me a menu to choose lunch. I suddenly felt sick and asked for just some peppermint tea. She said that I would have to wait a while and instead offered me more water to drink. I then fell asleep.

The same nurse returned with a pot of tea. An hour or so had passed. I had a sore throat developing which I was told commonly occurs after an operation. She gave me some tablets and asked if I would like anything to eat. I ordered an egg mayo sandwich. I did not want to risk more than that, although I had not eaten for many hours.

I lay there staring out of the window which overlooked a beautiful London bridge, my thoughts deep within my soul and, with all the will in the world, prayed for this to work.

I also started to wonder where Barry had disappeared to. He too had taken the day off work. I looked at my watch. It was lunchtime. He was probably feeding himself and drinking a beer or two at some local to calm his nerves.

My sandwich arrived. I was suddenly ravenous. So much so I asked for an extra round. My vocal chords were tightening up by then so I started to drink anything in sight. I knew also that I could only be released from hospital once I had urinated. I must have fallen asleep again, as the next thing I remember was Barry tapping me on the arm and asking how I was feeling.

He was jovial and nervous at the same time. He told me about his day. I was right in my previous assumption. He went to a great place for lunch and had a couple of beers. He browsed at shop windows, and just generally walked and walked to burn off excess nervous energy until he could walk no more. He reached the King's Road and then on to Sloane Square taking in the sights and sounds of London's fast-living. He said everything felt surreal as if he was in a dream. The reality of what we were doing suddenly hit him and he decided to return to me by bus. He had become physically and mentally tired but was excited and positive in his thinking.

I wish I could say I felt the same. I was just looking forward to going home and to feeling normal. Emotionally and physically I felt drained. All cleaned out! I knew this was far from over.

Finally, I did a couple of pees and it was time for the doctor to see me and advise me of what had taken place in the operation and to check me over. The lady fertilitist returned extremely pleased with what had been achieved and explained that the embryo transfer would take place in a couple of days.

Both Barry and I felt better for talking to her and she boosted our confidence, which was beginning to dip. She told me to get dressed, go home and to wait for a phone call from the laboratory to be informed of the results.

The next morning I knew as soon as the phone rang that it was the hospital. The bio-chemist informed me that we had been successful in that we had six very good embryos and that they had merged well.

Shortly after I received a call from a nurse confirming an appointment had been arranged. The transfer of the embryos from the dish to my insides was to take place the following morning.

I remember feeling excited and apprehensive all rolled into one that day. I remember it being a foggy morning. We walked over the bridge briskly as I had a very full and uncomfortable bladder. I had been instructed to drink plenty of water.

Later I found out the reason for this was so that an ultrasound scan could be performed simultaneously in order to view the position of the catheter being inserted during the transfer procedure.

It was a Saturday morning and so it was not too busy thankfully in the dreaded waiting room. We were shown to the room where I previously had the IUI performed.

I striped waist down and sat on the bed. A blanket was handed to me to cover the 'private parts'. I was told to slide my rear end towards the end of the bed so that my legs could be raised into the air and slip elegantly through the now famous stirrups.

Amazingly I felt calm and collected, so much so I hardly felt the cool gel smudged on my stomach for the ultrasound.

The screen placed on the wall in the top right hand-corner of that room flashed on and I stared at it waiting for something to appear. In unison the hatch beside the bed then screeched open and blobs appeared on the screen. I was shown the multitude of the embryos. Three were to be transferred from the six collected. (The law since has been changed so that only two can be transferred due to the dangers of multiple births.) The lab technician's outstretched arm emerged with her hand holding the priceless dish of embryos. The dish was passed over to the assisting nurse. The fertilitist inserted the embryos meticulously. It was like a smear test - no pain to speak of. The discomfort was the full bladder. I asked the question "Could I go for a pee quickly after the implementation"? The medical staff replied in unison "Yes". I was off that bed so quickly at the end of the procedure. I entered the ensuite bathroom. I could hear their voices through the door but that did not put me off. I had the longest pee with the biggest smile across my face and gave a huge sigh of relief. This was the best feeling in the whole wide world!

I got dressed and like before we were sent home with some pessaries which I had would have to insert either vaginally or rectally until the day of the pregnancy test. These pessaries were called Cyclogest. I also had been prescribed some other oral drugs to continue taking until further notice.

I had to take these in order to contain the hormone progesterone and to prepare the uterus for the ultimate. A pregnancy! Today was the 6 November 1999 - maybe my lucky number would be of help here (6 is my lucky number!)

As before, now came the difficult part. The nail-biting waiting time was upon us once again. Like before with the IUI we went immediately back to the daily grind of work for distraction.

Chapter Five

We were now in the gloomy month of November. It was typical for the time of year, plenty of grey drizzly English weather days. The brown dead damp leaves were truly driven into the ground.

A week had now passed since the insemination. It was Armistice weekend. We had the television on with the service from Horse Guards Cavalry drumming out their yearly tunes and marching music in the background whilst Barry and I were buried under a mountain of Sunday newspapers munching on some late breakfast. Like most people at that time of the year we needed a pick-me-up. I pinpointed a holiday amongst the many advertisements. We contemplated a weekend break to Europe half anticipating a failure on the IVF. We knew we were staying in London over Christmas/New Year as we wanted to be home for the Millennium celebrations.

We also concluded that since I would be doing a pregnancy test on a Saturday we would wait until the following day so as not to ruin the whole of next weekend. Do you really think we were that disciplined?

The following Saturday like clockwork as soon as I woke I did my bit in the bathroom as if it was just another day. I took out the pregnancy test from the bathroom cabinet remembering only too well from the last time what to expect or not to expect. To my utter amazement my heart missed a beat and I gulped putting my hand to my mouth to see that indeed there was a blue line the space within the window as it should be. I was pregnant. In total disbelief I did a double or maybe a triple take to check and see if I was not hallucinating. I then ran out to Barry and just pointed to the pregnancy test and said "take a look at that!"

He looked at me, smiled and said "Fantastic!" We then kissed, cuddled and jumped up and down with excitement. Our faces were continuously beaming. Neither of us held back. We were again two excited kids that had just opened the most amazing Christmas present.

We knew that we were far from being safely through the pregnancy itself and decided that we would hold back from telling people until we had passed the dangerous first three month trimester. My parents would be celebrating their wedding anniversary at the end of the week so we decided that with another week in hand, we would tell both sets of parents as they too were living through some of our anguish.

Barry and I came to the conclusion that November was not such a bad month after all that year, and the plans we had put forward the previous week were now discarded.

We excitedly told both sets of parents and my brother and sister-in-law. We went round with our bunch of flowers to my parents on their wedding anniversary and I swear even the flowers responded by living for an extra couple of weeks.

Whenever I paid a visit to the toilet, the habit of constantly looking to see if any blood had settled within my knickers would continue throughout that time and well into the pregnancy itself. I could not change the ingrained habit of looking to see if my period had arrived.

We went to the clinic to have the confirmation blood test, which was followed by the home pregnancy test. An early pregnancy scan on my sixth week of pregnancy had been arranged.

On arrival at the clinic we checked into reception with the biggest beaming smiles! We had only been sitting down a couple of minutes in the waiting room before the familiar smiling nurse greeted us with hugs and congratulations.

She took us into the familiar box room for my confirmation blood test, proving that indeed I was pregnant.

We were then told to sit in the waiting room directly outside the scan analyst's office. The analyst who checked over the contents of the scan confirmed that indeed there was one healthy sac. She pointed out to me a grainy blob on the screen; however, I was honestly none the wiser from seeing what was on screen. A copy was printed and to this day I still proudly retain.

The scan analyst had become a familiar face throughout the scans that had taken place during the IVF treatment itself. So when she had the pleasant job of confirming that indeed I was pregnant, the feelings of joy expressed were sincere. We said our farewells because as she reminded me I was about to embark on my next journey of pregnancy with new consultants elsewhere. In other words, I now was being redirected on to the normal route of pregnancy.

We were told to keep in contact with the clinic and to inform them of our progress. We thanked the familiar staff and bid our farewells.

I made an appointment with my GP to inform him of the pregnancy and at the same time I rang the hospital where I wanted to have the baby, for an appointment arranging for my introduction to an obstetrician and for an opening scan.

This was indeed a happy time. We were walking on air! We thought what a start to the new millennium. We were at long last to be a Mummy & Daddy. Our heritage would live on. I would be a Mummy at 40! No better birthday gift. The gift of life!

Barry's parents lived in Nottingham so we broke the good news on a marathon of a phone call and the promise of informing them of progress at Christmas in person.

Christmas had already been previously arranged that I was doing the whole caboodle and I enthusiastically insisted on still making it but now as a double celebration for all of us.

A week or so later morning sickness kicked in (all-day in fact) but I did not have a care in the world. Difficult or not I was going to do the Christmas celebration. I wanted this baby and all the baggage that comes with being pregnant. Nothing was going to stop me now. I was on a mission!

Generally I was sensible. Not that we had a huge social life at that time but we did pretty much become couch potatoes. I felt tired and extremely sore from the injection scars which had left my body very bruised. I had a constant metallic taste in my mouth which I had been told is the "pregnancy sign" but I am sure it was also the backlash from the bombardment of drugs I had swallowed and injected. The last thing I wanted to do was go out and eat or drink in public with the chances of vomiting in some cubby-hole of a loo.

This was to be the best Christmas ever. I was a child all over again. With the little energy I had I surpassed myself and walked up and down the shopping malls with a smile at everyone, buying for as many people as I could. I was probably more extravagant that year than most due to the fact I was having the best present of all. The future looked rosy. Our new baby, in the years to come, would be part of the forthcoming celebration and many other family occasions.

At long last maybe I would be accepted and not shunned as the barren relative or friend. People often think they are being kind by being not in your face on children's party invites or special outings. In retrospect this in fact has the opposite affect. We were being alienated, made to feel totally worthless and of no importance, because we did not have offspring. I know that other childless couples have also experienced this wavelength.

It would have been more acceptable to have been asked or if people had been upfront and not hush-hushed behind closed doors. It only added to the feeling of inadequacy and made one feel even more isolated. It was more hurtful or even pathetic to find out through third parties of our exclusion. We had to live with it. We were being excluded from one of the most basic routines of life. Watch our child grow!

We sent birthday cards, gifts and congratulations. Sometimes we would be invited as an afterthought. That was fine, and then at least we were given the option of acceptance or declining as adults and not imbeciles. We were human beings who just could not have children!

As time went by eventually it was clear this was one of the reasons we would lose more and more friends. They were uncomfortable and in between the lines we were made to feel we had nothing in common. 'Ps and Qs' were being watched from both sides.

As pleased as we were for our family members and friends we still felt we would never have the inclusion returned. The pain was sometimes intolerable. To most it seemed this did not exist. We felt we did not belong to the most exclusive club. We were in no-mans land. People thought they were doing us a kindness in their exclusion to save us from the pain of what we were missing out on. The bottom line is that there is no right or wrong. There was no escape. We could not produce a child. We took it for granted that we would be allocated God's gift. The hurt anger and pain is just all rolled into one for the barren couple!

Christmas day arrived as it always does on a damp drizzly mild day. We saw no children making snowmen, or sledging in the snow outside through our rain dripped windows.

As normal, the family arrived at lunchtime to a rather ashen and nauseous chef. We opened our gifts which had been piled in the corner of the room looking like a mini Mount Everest.

We were all talking about the baby. Which room in our house was to be the nursery, colour schemes and trying to guess which sex with a selection of names and having bets as to when exactly it would be born. We even produced the scan picture which we passed around with all of us not having a clue of what we were really looking at.

Barry served lunch as I became extremely queasy. The last thing I fancied doing was to serve an avalanche of food. The smell of that lunch is still with me to this day. There was no way I could have served it up on to the table without heaving.

I made my excuses and went upstairs to have a lie down with many happy thoughts of plans to be put into operation. Spilling out from downstairs the laughter was jovial and apparent. I was sure it was one of my father-in-law's jokes. As soon as the sickness passed my intention was to return to that very happy room.

I could not wait for the year 2000 to roll in. I would also be starting my third month of pregnancy.

We decided that we would wait until the first three months had passed before announcing to friends and work colleagues our good news. We had been married at that stage over five years so we agreed that an announcement could wait another few weeks. It was to be a special year in more ways than one!

Chapter Six

*T*he millennium celebrations came and went pretty much as most New Years Eves. We went out with some friends over dinner. Booze was out of the question for me but Barry and the others enjoyed getting truly bamboozled. I was elected as the taxi driver for that night/morning.

In my mind I did plenty of praying that evening that everything should go to plan for the Year 2000! It was to be my 40th birthday in June and to have a new son or daughter in July.

Personally, since the beginning of December it had been a trying time for me as I felt sick 24-hours a day. Sometimes there would be a respite during the evening for a couple of hours but the dreadful metallic taste would linger. So much so that although I am generally a chocoholic at this time I could only face eating fruit, which I found refreshing and quite a contrast from the usual; salads were also a favourite at that time. I was sure that I would not be the first anorexic mother. Realistically, this was no time for diets!

I spoke to my GP who reassured me that many people do get day sickness and not just morning and that during the next trimester I would regain a huge appetite. Relax, chill-out, enjoy!

Work was plentiful at the beginning of January and pretty much occupied most of my time. I was busy arranging, on behalf of a large corporation, their hospitality for the forthcoming Rugby Union fixtures. I remember this well as it was a French client who had travelled to London and I had to meet him over lunch in the West End. It was hard to be focused as I was extremely nauseous and as much as it was a worthwhile meeting, I reckon I was too often in the toilet wondering if I was actually going to vomit. I never did.

I had also received many enquiries for the many forthcoming summer events so thankfully I was kept busy generally; working in my office in the safe haven of home and not forced to use public loos.

The next couple of weeks in January passed very peacefully in as much I had my six week scan (on the seventh week - a week later due to the Christmas break), which to our delight we witnessed seeing a white blob flashing on and off (heartbeat) placed in the centre of the placenta. It was confirmed that there was indeed one baby and we were told that at our next scan we could be told the sex of the baby if we wanted to satisfy our curiosity.

I remember not long after having that scan that I physically began to feel more human. The bruising from the IVF was fast disappearing and I started to have more of an appetite for food. In fact, looking back I felt bloody marvellous, especially for January. The nausea was subsiding. I had the odd headache, but counted my lucky stars I did not have flu. I did not wish to invade my body with any more drugs if I could help it.

During the last week of December I had a mini-scare in as much as I had stomach cramps like period pains and the odd drop of blood for a couple of days. This was called spit-spotting and I was reassured by the GP that this was common. Many pregnant women would often bleed within their first few months of pregnancy but continue to have a child as the end result.

I also rang the fertility clinic who also confirmed that unless the bleeding became more definite in its colour and the actual amount deposited, there was nothing too much to worry about.

The cramps did disappear as did the bleeding. I felt fine even to the point that I now had very little morning sickness.

The following couple of weeks after that I continued as normal. On 19 January, I was at my desk typing an invoice when I suddenly got the most horrendous stomach cramp. It was late morning, around lunchtime.

To my utter despair I visited the loo only to discover that I was bleeding once again but more heavily than a couple of weeks previously. I was literally shaking like a leaf trying to hold back all my anxieties of the moment. So much so, I did not know who to call first. In between frequent visits to the loo I plucked the courage to ring the fertility clinic first, who advised me to ring my OB or GP in order that a scan could be arranged.

I then rang my GP who was not around but I was advised by the receptionist that he would be back later in the afternoon. I told her of my urgency and became emotional. She suggested that I went directly to the local hospital for a scan but also hinted that there could be a long wait. Knowing the hospital, I too knew that it could be a long wait. I had waited too long to be pregnant; I was not about to wait too long to be told I am not pregnant.

I went back to the loo and had another peak. The bleeding had slightly subsided so maybe this was a false alarm. I rang my OB who suggested I go privately along to Harley Street to have a scan. He would make an appointment on my behalf for two o'clock that afternoon. I did not care what it cost I just wanted to get this sorted.

I rang for a taxi for practical reasons. There was no way I wanted to get stuck in a traffic jam or have problems parking. I wanted to avoid as much as stress as possible.

Once seated in the taxi I started to relax as much as I could to answer politely to the cabby's continuous banter. The good thing was that it did take my mind off things. I arrived at the scanning clinic and I waited my turn more relaxed than I had been during the previous hour.

I remember chatting merrily to the scan operator who in turn was asking how things had been since the last scan. I told her that I had felt good during the last couple of weeks.

The scan I was about to have was external. The cool gel was splashed across my stomach. She pursued with more pleasantries and then she became very quiet. How I remember that! I asked her if everything was alright. She then told me she was going to call on someone else to assist and would return in a minute. As quick as she left the room another woman assisted and together they looked at the screen intensely. The first lady then very directly told me that they could not find a heartbeat and that judging by the size of the foetus it had died on my 11th week. I was now mid-way through my 13th week so the foetus had been dead for the last fortnight or so. They told me that I would have to undergo an operation under anaesthetic which is called a D&C (Dilation and Curettage) whereby the remains from conception are scraped out. They asked who my OB was and where I would like this to happen!

I just sat up on the bed looking at the screen but nothing would come out of my lips. I was in shock! They then asked if they should call Barry.

I was in denial as I asked again if they were absolutely sure that I had indeed miscarried. I could not grasp the diagnosis as I reiterated that I had felt fine over the last couple of weeks.

The waterworks then started to flow and I balled my eyes out like a newborn baby. Through my sobs I rang Barry on the mobile. I knew that he had a high profile meeting that day so I had disturbed him with what had been going on to add to his stresses and strains of the day. As it turned out he was out at a business lunch.

He did not quite comprehend what I was telling him and was trying to ascertain my whereabouts. To him I was not making sense. He made his excuses to his clients and exited swiftly to his car in a confused state.

After the scan I hurriedly got dressed. Wiping away my tears, I was told to wait in the reception area while the scanners would telephone my OB. They spoke to him and it had been arranged that since his practice was only two doors down the street Barry and I were to meet with him. I had told Barry to meet me there at the OB's reception area and to take his time by driving safely.

Do not ask me how but I held it together, even when I first saw Barry who was ashen faced repeatedly asking "Why, Why, Why?"

We went and saw our OB promptly whereby he reconfirmed what the two radiologists had previously told me. I was to have the D&C immediately. He told us that I would be staying overnight at a well-known West End Hospital. I checked in there and then, and could not eat any food due to the anaesthetic being administered for the operation, and hence the reason for the overnight stay.

Barry drove us to the hospital which was only a short drive away. I remember it having a plush reception area and seeing someone well-known walk pass me with their new bundle of joy. It is a well-known hospital for that type of clientele to have their babies delivered at. It was inevitable, as I sarcastically commented to Barry, that today of all days we would even do this in style. If you ask me today who that person was, I just cannot remember as to be frank I was numb. We both were. Little did we know the best was yet to come!

I was eventually checked in and repeatedly I had to sign one form after another also because this I was told could be claimed on our medical insurance. Thank god for small mercies! (No sympathy was shown by the insurers as we were slightly late in paying and they were on our backs like a ton of bricks.)

Barry went back home with my list of requirements. I must admit I do not remember too much of that evening since I had to blank it out in order not to become hysterical that night.

The following morning was very much a similar routine to what I undergone for the IVF. The only difference now was that they were removing the baby instead of inserting one. I did ask if there was anything to see of the baby and was told that there would be nothing recognisable to view. So we would never find out its sex.

Although I was now in a different hospital the procedures were exactly the same. I had my blood pressure taken, body temperature reading and I was introduced to the anaesthetist who explained the procedure. My OB also was close at hand to answer any questions I had.

Like before, the attendees arrived on cue and I was ushered down on the mobile bed through the cold antiseptic corridors leading to the theatre. God this was bleak! No jokes offered by the medical staff this time! It was just a countdown before being unconscious.

I woke up back in a mini-ward with about three other patients to recuperate. I just wanted to sleep as I was so thoroughly dejected.

I was told that I would be able to leave during the afternoon after I had passed urine and eaten. I was given some oral medication and was told to continue once at home. The pain and bleeding would continue similar to that of a period. A scan and blood test would be taken a week later as confirmation that all was clear.

As it turned out I went for the confirmation scan/blood test on the 26 January only to be told that I was not clear and that I would have to go through the whole operation again. I was angry, upset and truly devastated that this was to be carried out on the following day at the same hospital.

Barry wanted to sue the operatives but I told him I was beyond that and all I wanted to do was get the whole task in hand over and done with and to forget the painful saga. He honoured that and probably, in hindsight, it was the best move we made.

We checked in that day and the procedures were identical to what I had undergone only a week earlier. It was shit! My mood was hostile. It was not surprising with all the hormones raging as well as dealing with the obvious!

To top it all it took forever to be discharged on that stay and I was kept over for an extra night as a cautionary view due to feeling extremely nauseous for longer than I should have.

Once I was released, Barry told me that he had met someone he knew through work in the hospital lift. She was visiting her sister with her mother. She had the biggest smile across her face and questioned Barry as to what reason he was at the hospital. Before Barry could reply, she excitedly proceeded to announce that her sister had just given birth. Barry replied that he was visiting me and told them that I had undergone a miscarriage. The facial expression changed from both women and the lift became silent. So much so, nothing more was said, not even goodbye when they all departed.

The following week I had to undergo yet another scan and blood test before being given the all clear.

The devastation of what we had lost began to sink in and it was a miserable February. Barry and I decided that we were most certainly taking a break from all the emotional and physical trials and tribulations of fertility treatment.

I could no longer face the constant intake of drugs. The only pills I continued to take were the folic acid tablets which can prevent spina bifida. At my age I felt it was vital to take these. I was always encouraged to take this before trying to become pregnant.

We were both racked with grief, remorse and anger. In my quiet moments I would often bury my head amongst the pillows of our bed and consistently punch the pillows with all the pent up frustration and eventually burying my face into them sobbing. I cried and cried until no more tears could pour out. We had lost our baby and the baby had lost its quest for life. All our dreams had been shattered and even then that was not straight-forward. It bloody hurt.

We had received a letter from the fertility clinic informing us that there was a support group for miscarriages which we could attend during that time or in the future.

We decided at that stage to deal with the dilemma of the loss ourselves but I did keep their details on file.

Chapter Seven

It was now time to take time off from the rollercoaster ride of fertility treatment. Nothing would fill the void of the miscarriage itself but Barry and I knew that we had to move on or we would be totally eaten up. We had achieved what we thought was becoming more and more unlikely. I had actually conceived and by becoming pregnant we now knew that there was a possibility of falling pregnant again. We had to take the positive from the hand we had been dealt.

We decided that it was now time to go it alone. We would shag this way, that way and anyway we could, and enjoy it! The full moon played its part. Upside down, legs left high against the wall, and at different times of the day. We were now free. No specific times to adhere to. In other words, no fertility tracking system. We were back to using our aromatherapy oils in twinkling candlelight! We had forgotten how to enjoy a truly good bonk! It was time to have fun. We went on holiday to my brother's home in

Florida and became more refreshed and revitalised; the weight had been lifted from our shoulders but this was only to be temporary.

We had two further courses of IVF treatment that year. The first was on 23 June the day before my 40th birthday. This course proved to be the least successful as seven oocytes (eggs) were collected and only two were good quality hence only two embryos were good enough to be transferred into my uterus.

The second course of treatment followed on the 26 October, when nine oocytes were collected, four of good quality but as the ruling was at that time only three embryos could be transferred.

Outsiders to this sort of treatment are probably wondering why I would put myself through this so quickly after having the miscarriage at the beginning of the year and with the subsequent no-go of the June IVF.

The reasons were because we were quite simply up against the clock and we were also told that our best chances were whilst we were undergoing the constant use of fertility drugs.

Looking back, certainly from the second course of IVF, this did not prove to be the case.

By the end of that year I was physically and mentally all cleaned out! It was time to go away and have a bloody good re-think. Christmas was on its way and no way on earth did I want to relive the memories from the previous year. We felt we deserved a well earned holiday and to just disappear to somewhere with a golden sunset.

We added up our finances and unfortunately for us we just did not have enough money to go around. We counted our blessings that at least we were giving it a bloody good go on the IVF front.

With help from my brother and our building society accounts, we were fortunately able to give ourselves the chances. On the NHS this would not have applied.

The holiday was put on the back burner. We somehow muddled through Christmas and the New Year celebrations but as anticipated expressed now and again our apathy of what had been going on over the past year.

The year 2001 rolled in. Barry and I had the opportunity to attend The World Sports Awards at the Royal Albert Hall on 16 January 2001. We were to stay at the London Hilton Hotel in Park Lane with a party being given the night before for Muhammad Ali's 59th birthday party. It included a two-night stay in a suite at the Hotel with all its comforts, accompanied by the most fabulous views over London.

Those two days were just what the doctor ordered. We lost ourselves. We were in a world of well-known faces, successful people in their field with many interesting stories to tell. They were achievers in chasing and acting out their dreams.

At the party we were put on a table of sports journalists from all over the world and got truly sozzled. We saw one recognisable boxer after another and many well-known sports personalities. It was very surreal. We even got close to the great man himself who was surrounded by amicable boxers and bodyguards. For Barry and I being true sports buffs - this was a dream come true.

The following evening we dolled ourselves up once again to attend the awards at the Royal Albert Hall. We entered the building via the red carpet treatment which was fun as we could overhear the watching crowd holding their autograph books with pen enclenched, whispering "who are those two?"

I remember after the awards had been presented, we travelled in a coach from the Royal Albert Hall back to the hotel in order to attend an after-show party.

The atmosphere of the party was great. Ice statues were elevated all around the room. Music was blaring with plenty of energetic dancing. Magicians doing their party tricks. Titbits were being served to eat accompanied by plenty of champers.

Linford Christie and I were having a race with cocktail sticks as to which of us could find the most mango and orange melon chunks.

I even met Arsene Wenger which, for me as a Gunner's fan, was the absolute! Barry got to meet Lennox Lewis which for him was his ultimate.

It was pure escapism and a real uplift in January for both of us. Thank god I took the camera with! The only bad bit about those two nights away was the fact that I was menstruating. Bloody typical!

The following morning we were on the most almighty high of what had taken place during those last couple of days. We knew there and then it was very special.

Whilst having a delicious breakfast that morning, I had the opportunity of speaking to the greatest Olympic swimmer of them all, Mark Spitz (he won seven gold medals at the 1972 Olympic Games) and I made a complete arse of myself by saying that I too was a Champion swimmer. The words came out wrong. When I was 10 at school I became champion at backstroke within the borough of Westminster. Not quite the same, is it!

February became our discussion month. We were at loose ends. We were not sure which direction to take.

The good thing was that I had a good turnover at work that month and Barry also had pulled off some deals. We decided to make an appointment with the fertility clinic director to try and find out what, if anything, we could do to make our chances better. We knew that with the race against time we had to act quickly and also before our morale would turn totally negative. We had to be positive.

We had a 1.30pm appointment arranged for Thursday 15 March at the fertility clinic. We were greeted by the familiar faces at the reception area and like true experts we trooped into the waiting room but instead of staring at the gloomy faces we decided to bury ourselves in some office paperwork. We were right to do so; once again we were kept waiting longer than we should have been. A good hour later we were collected by a nurse and shown to the fertilitist's office.

To my surprise, as I am the more outspoken, Barry took the reins. Barry very directly complained that we were spending, spending, spending but had a 'no go' on the IUI, a miscarriage on our first IVF, and two more IVF cycles which just did not connect. In short we had already had four cycles - resulting in nothing except depleted money resources. How could he help? What were we to do? Did they know why it was not working? Age and time were progressing. Would we ever be parents through the IVF procedures?

His answer in the main was that we should just keep on trying. I intercepted and asked how long and how many times would the clinic expect us to continue. He truthfully answered: "No one knows, as I told you before you come under the category of inexplicable circumstances. Many couples have gone through treatments many more times than you have already. Some become pregnant, others don't."

Obviously the fact that I was now coming up to 41 put us also in the higher band of less probable but at the same time my eggs did not seem to be a problem and were generally of good quality.

He did suggest that if we put ourselves on a waiting list for donated eggs from a younger donor our percentages would also become better, but in the next breath he told us that no guarantee could be given. The list had a backlog of a year to 18 months at that point in time. The cost for this service would be £100.

He did also suggest that he would change some of the drug regimes within the cycle.

We concluded our meeting by informing him that we would mull over what had just been discussed. Easter was on its way and since it had been a long time since we had been away we wanted time to digest the information and discuss it in relaxed surroundings. We needed to recharge our batteries. We were exhausted from putting in extra hours at work to make ends meet, together with the added strain from all the treatment we had already undergone. We would confirm on our return whether or not we wished to go ahead with any further treatment.

By the time we reached Florida that Easter we were totally flunked. My period had just started as had so often been the case whenever I took a holiday. Whether it was a long weekend break or a fortnight, you can bet my monthly accompanist would join the visit!

It was a 10 day break which we decided would be dedicated as to which direction we should now take and at the same time to do absolutely zilch.

The weather was fabulous and our pale complexions began to change to a much healthier look. We lay outstretched wearing our sunshades, smothered in the latest Hawaiian Tropic oils, our skins glistening in the sunlight. We were gazing upwards admiring the blue sky watching a small aircraft cut out through its tail-end marking the sky by way of sending out heart shaped messages of "I Love You". Our huge sun loungers were set side by side by the pool, and we quenched our thirst by sipping long cool drinks bulging with ice cubes in pint size glasses, dipping in and out of the refreshing swimming pool, agreeing and disagreeing over several points of the matter in hand.

We also had many laughs on this holiday. We witnessed a middle-aged American couple have a real rant in a restaurant for a good half an hour or so. It was so funny that we had tears in our eyes from all the laughter. It could not have been acted out better in a Hollywood film.

Whilst queuing at the many restaurant outlets waiting to be seated at our table, we got to talk to every Tom, Dick and Harry and I swear that every American we met asked: "Do you know … they live in London?" There was another remark that had us in stitches. "Oh you are English not Australian. Australia is the next country to you isn't it!" and "Is England part of London?"

We nearly missed the flight home as we got lost finding the drop-off location for the rental car.

The day before we left we came jointly to the decision that we would give the IVF run another go on our return. Time was of the essence here. We both believed that whilst we were fit and positive in our thinking, we had to go ahead quickly and precisely, instead of dawdling on waiting lists. Both our commissions from work would be in the bank on our return. The money was there; we had to gamble. It was baby lottery time!

On our return I was booked in to have the ultrasound scan and to have our follow up consultation. All was well and I would start again with the nasal spray at the end of April. Here we go again!

Chapter Eight

*I*t is strange sometimes how the human mind plays its part. I felt very positive about the next course of treatment. We returned from holiday and literally started the treatment with immediate effect.

My mother and father-in-law were to celebrate their 50th wedding anniversary. They lived in Nottingham and we set off up the M1 to join their celebration with friends and family who we had not seen in a while.

It was a bright, cool sunny day on the last day of April. Barry and I looked tanned and healthy. We were, as always, greeted with such love. We were asked if we had a good holiday and then came the onslaught of questions about our conception plans.

It was the same at all social gatherings, whether it was with family or friends. I would always be prepared with some responses for people that would insist on asking "when are you going to start a family?" "Don't leave it too late." "Sorry to hear about the miscarriage but try again you will be wonderful parents."

Inevitably some people say things that seem thoughtless and uncaring but they have little understanding of infertility or what we were going through. So either I chose not to respond or I would keep explanations brief and factual knowing that their comprehension was unlikely.

We enjoyed the celebration and wished bon voyage to Barry's parents who were about to fulfil one of their lifetime dreams as passengers on the cruise liner QE2.

During May I visited the clinic for a routine scan to check that everything was OK to commence with the bombardment of the fertility injections.

Before sleeping it became a nightly routine for Barry to confidently administer the intra-muscular injections. I would become tense, apprehensive, even ratty, whilst I watched him ensure that no air got into the catheter. He would slowly ensure that there were no air bubbles showing within the dosage by flicking the sides of the catheter itself. In the beginning, even though the nurse had shown him the method, he had been paranoid that he would mess up and cause me pain but with encouragement and reassurance from me, his confidence grew over time and he became quicker at the job.

Although I would now openly admit that I detested it and, yes, it did hurt. I would close my eyes and grit my teeth with clenched fists as I felt the needle jut its way into my flabby flesh. It was a quick pinch but afterwards I would feel sore and would bruise black and blue for months. I flinch now just thinking about it. I hated needles then and I hate them now!

On the 6 June 2001 it most definitely was D Day. It was the day I had been booked in for my egg collection. This was becoming boring; I knew the routine too well.

I was waiting to be knocked out by the anaesthetist; once she arrived she introduced herself and seemed to know who I was. Apparently she was a close friend of the lady fertilitist that had been around when I had been successfully pregnant. I had obviously made some impression.

She was chatting to me like a long-lost friend asking me where I lived, what I do for a living, could I get her tickets, did I have a pet. That is the god's honest truth. Eventually she did knock me out in more ways than one!

When I woke up after the operation, I remember her saying that I "had done brilliantly by producing eleven fabulous eggs". There was no let-off from this woman.

It was back to the waiting game in and out of the clinic. The good thing though was that it was June and there were plenty of distractions at that time of the year.

It so happened that my birthday, 24 June, was the day allocated as the pregnancy test day. We were tempted to delay it by a day to avoid any disappointment but we agreed we had to continue in the pattern of positive thinking! It could be a wonderful birthday present, the best!

The night before my birthday we went out and had an enjoyable dinner with plenty of laughter at Quaglino's, a well-known restaurant in the West End, with another couple for a joint birthday celebration.

The following morning I woke up to an array of flowers and a mountain of birthday cards. A breakfast tray was laid across my lap against the duvet. It was a Sunday morning and Barry insisted that today I was to have a lie in before, at my own pace, doing the pregnancy test. Breakfast was delicious, with pancakes and seasonal fruits accompanied by a mug of hot chocolate.

I digested my food and went back to reading the cards together with the Sunday newspapers, just like it was any other Sunday.

During mid-morning I got out of bed with all fingers crossed. I did my knicker check first to see if any blood had arrived. It hadn't. This was a good sign. I took a deep breath and opened the packet of testers. I did my pee trying to catch the stick and praying for this all to be worthwhile. I waited the allocated time for the result. Sure enough in the window appeared a very prominent blue line. I jumped for joy and punched the air, shouting "Yes". I said to myself I am going to be positive ... positive ... positive. It is going to work this time.

I sent out a cat-cry to Barry informing him of the news. He responded by rushing up the stairs in order to give me the biggest bear hug and excitedly said that he was booking lunch somewhere for the two of us to celebrate.

I rang the clinic the following morning to arrange the confirmation blood test together with a scan. They told me to give it 10 days so that a scan could be performed. This would be shortly before we were to travel on a pre-arranged a holiday to Greece. The appointment was made for Thursday 5 July.

I was given the go ahead - everything was fine and as it should be. I was definitely pregnant. We had a busy weekend scheduled. We were attending the Madonna concert on the Saturday night and going to the Wimbledon final on Sunday and travelling out on Monday. We came to the decision to cut out the concert and just attend Wimbledon. Luck was neither on our side that day nor Tim Henman's. Instead of seeing the pre-scheduled final we saw the semi-final whereby Tim lost his overnight lead against Goran Ivanisivic and we saw instead a predictable Ladies final with Venus Williams winning. The Men's final was to be moved to the following day. We were unable to watch it as in Greece it was not part of their television schedule.

We went outside Centre Court to the surrounding areas and sat and had a coffee when suddenly I said to Barry I had stomach cramps and that I wanted to do a knicker check. He told me to relax and that everything will be OK. I went to the public toilets nonetheless.

I could not quite believe it and continued to be in slight denial but sure enough there was a small puddle of blood soaked within the knickers.

I returned to the table where I had left Barry and told him that we should make tracks back home. He understood without any words spoken as to the reason why.

We returned home disappointed but were relieved that we had pre-packed our suitcases all ready to go in the morning. After eating later that evening the bleeding had definitely eased. I experienced slight cramps but it was nothing too untoward.

We discussed whether or not we should cancel the holiday but jointly agreed it was early days. We were aware that spit-spotting can occur in early pregnancy. It was Sunday, so who would we have called? We spoke briefly to the fertility clinic who offered us the same advice. If I was to lose the baby it would run its own course and the best place to recuperate would be on holiday. Also the bleed had virtually stopped by bedtime. It probably was a false alarm. I was tired and preventing any emotion from surfacing; we both were.

Early the following morning, the first thing I did was an anxious knicker check. All was fine. Thank God!

At the airport to be on the safe side I bought sanitary products. I was still not 100% convinced. I felt as if a period was on its way but during the whole of the fertility treatment you feel crampy as well as crappy.

When we did check in at the B.A. desk at Gatwick we were told that our flight to Athens had been delayed and that we were to transfer by coach to Heathrow. Barry told them that I was in early pregnancy and that it was stress we could well have done without.

He raised the question as to why we did not receive notification before leaving home. They apologised and said that we were well within the time limits in order to catch the new allocated flight.

Our trek on the M25 was a quiet one although the same could not be said of the traffic that morning. We decided to stay chilled. It was the best way; what would be, would be.

We made the flight and had a smooth journey in the skies. We were greeted by our courier who took us to the familiar hotel that we had been going to for years. We felt like we were home from home. We checked into the hotel and relaxed for the remainder of that day. I did not move other than to go down for dinner. We were feverishly searching for the tennis final on the television in the room but in the end we opted for the easier route. We tracked down the result by the internet link on our mobiles. We knew we had missed a classic.

Everything from that point went further downhill, a lot further. The following morning I woke up to a pool of blood smeared on me and the bed sheets. The worse scenario had occurred. We had lost the baby.

Communication was difficult from where we were and eventually the clinic returned my call. I calmly took on board what they were telling me. They told me to expect the situation to be similar to that of an ordinary period but I may bleed more heavily and the duration would be longer. I should take paracetamol to ease the cramps should there be any. There would be no need for me to have a D&C this time round as it was only just six weeks into the pregnancy and everything would dissolve. I was booked in for an ultrasound on my return. Great!

By the time we got back there was no blood in sight. I had bled for the first 10 days of my holiday, duly cleaned out. I had a cry on the first day but we decided we were on holiday and it obviously was not meant to be. Life goes on. We would ask the questions when we got back. We needed answers and we knew we couldn't get them in Greece.

I must be honest - the miscarriage did not hinder me too much. I was numb from it. My mindset was as if I just had another period that went on for longer than normal.

Coincidently, a close friend of mine was also on holiday in a different part of Greece at the same time as us. She had experienced a miscarriage and unluckily for her she had to undergo a D&C in Greece in some decrepid hospital. This was because she was further down the road than me. About eight weeks pregnant. She certainly did not recommend it! I only found out her sad news on our return from holiday, as we had not been in communication whilst out there.

The best tonic for Barry and I on our return was to go out and enjoy ourselves! It was mid-July and sumptuously warm, continental-like. We attended a fabulous open air concert at Hyde Park the following weekend linking up with plenty of eating, drinking and being merry. Too much sadness had gone by and no doubt there was plenty more to come.

Chapter Nine

Once again I cancelled all the arrangements I had made pre-holiday with the hospital where I intended to have the baby delivered. I also spoke to my new obstetrician and informed him that his services would not be required with regard to delivering the baby we so desired.

He recommended that we should continue trying and that he would have no hesitation in recommending this specific fertility clinic to us or someone else in a similar situation, classed as "inexplicable". We were, as far as he was concerned, at the right place to handle our situation.

He had received a letter from the fertility clinic informing him of our disappointing news. He asked to be kept informed of our plans and if he could be of help he would be there for us.

I went to the fertility clinic and had an ultrasound scan to confirm that indeed I had lost the baby. No sac was showing and all had been flushed out naturally.

At the same time we had a follow-up with a consultant who confirmed that there had been ovarian cysts/fibroids present but could not confirm whether or not that was the reason for the miscarriage. I asked what preventive methods could be utilised. He responded that fibroids grow as the pregnancy develops and that it is quite normal. He then proceeded to ask if we required any counselling for the loss that we had suffered and if we had any plans to try again.

I calmly (although I wanted to scream at him, there was nothing wrong with my head) responded that both of us were totally bemused with the situation and we were getting on with life the best way we could, and as we had previously.

I also said that we were unsure what direction to pursue. I felt that my body had taken enough punishment internally and externally and that I wanted to take time out. I also said bluntly "we had already lost enough money for nothing, it just does not grow on trees". In short we did not want to be bullied into taking another course of IVF treatment. Funds were simply not available. Were they offering?!

Before the end of the meeting I agreed to make an appointment with the counsellor within the clinic for both of us.

The following week we attended the meeting and both of us expressed our desolate feelings about the emotional, physical and financially demanding times that we had already undertaken to no avail.

During this meeting we told the lady counsellor that it is very hard to express the emotional experience to people that have not gone through it themselves. We felt that we were victims of life itself and that we were grieving for ourselves as if we had been faced with our own deaths. Our family line for both of us was to cease existing. As a couple we had been strong and felt that we had grown closer through the trials and tribulations.

We talked of our helplessness and the personally upsetting and irritating experiences that we had faced; the feelings of jealousy, sadness and resentment when facing child-centred attractions or events; watching parents' relationships with their offspring; disliking or admiring their behaviour and attitudes towards their children. The loneliness and exclusions of not being a parent. We were drifting away from friends as we were losing common ground. The thoughtless and uncaring or insensitive remarks often made but unintended.

We also talked along the lines of adoption, whether we could live with that and to discuss that option as a possibility in the future.

She concluded the meeting, saying that she thought that we were both well-balanced and seemed to be dealing with the trilogy of fertility treatment. None of the remarks we had expressed were unusual to any other couple in the same predicament. If we wanted to bleed our hearts further we could call her at any time or she could recommend a specialist group outside of the clinic.

We thanked her for her advice and left the clinic talking about adoption. We had not volunteered to go down that road when we first started getting involved with fertility treatment, and we had not discussed it since those early days.

Arrogantly we had always assumed eventually we would be parents naturally, even if it meant via fertility experiments. The apple was just not there to be picked off the tree. We needed time to digest what had just taken place.

The talk benefited us temporarily. I did some research and phoned different adoption agencies and found out what route one had to take in order to become accepted on the list for adopting a child. The process seemed to be very long and drawn out and, like everything else, not necessarily straightforward. I was asked very personal questions and felt that it was too much hard work with my frame of mind at that time. The age cut-off point appeared to be 45 but did vary from agency to agency.

Barry was more negative than me about pursuing this avenue and hence it did not take too much to dampen my spirit.

I was banging my head against a brick wall. I was sure that the mood swings were caused by the huge intake of all the fertility drugs. The hormones were raging. I know I was hell to live with.

After a couple of months, my obsession with being a parent was causing me more anguish than ever before. Anger was beginning to surface from both of us. Tempers would be raised far more easily than normal, even for the most trivial of things. The frustration that what we had been pursuing was looking more and more like a fantasy and not reality.

I felt like I was losing control of my identity. The feeling of despair and loss began to take over. I started to worry about the damage to my health, body and sanity one moment and in the next not giving a damn. I was beginning to become very conscious of my age and appearance and feeling frustrated that the clock could not be turned back. I also felt that as much as our lovemaking was not on a fertility clock we were still up against the clock of life.

I was even more sensitive to being out in public; whether it was a shopping centre, parking lot or park watching mummies push their child's buggy with such haste. I found it difficult to be in the company of friends with their children on full view going through the motions accordingly.

Tears would often flow at an instant more than previously. I was very tearful, I was unhappy, I was unfulfilled, I was lonely, I was jealous, I was frightened, I was angry, I was in mourning. Conclusion: I was depressed.

Even through the haze of my depression I knew that Barry was also suffering and often we would just say nothing and have a good old-fashioned hug. There were no words that could fulfil the emptiness we endured.

If you have been there you understand; if you have not then to you it will be incomprehensible that people strive so much to have a baby.

People like myself, who have undergone fertility treatment year in year out and who would dearly love to attain God's gift naturally, will always understand, whether they eventually are successful in their pursuit or not.

However, some of us are not so lucky and have had to settle for no children or have taken other options that are permissible, whether it be adoption, surrogacy or fostering. Those were the options before we became fortunate to live within an era whereby artificial insemination is widely available (even though currently still based on percentages) - albeit whether one has to pay privately or, if you are really fortunate, via the NHS treatment scheme.

What I did learn throughout the experience was that nothing should ever be taken for granted. Like most things in life you have to strive for it. You either strike lucky or you don't.

As difficult as it was, the percentages were highly stacked against us.

Yes, today there is the advantage of freezing eggs whether it is ones own or donated. Together with improving technology the medical field are making discoveries and always going forward, the whole problem of conceiving and holding onto a baby may well change. Maybe even become obsolete. I am not a doctor, I do not know.

However, the human attitude is that it will not happen to me but to some other poor bugger. So the idea immediately becomes an afterthought. Do not let this happen if you can prevent it. It really hurts - all the time!

So how does one get on with life and rid oneself of the pain of being barren? If someone out there knows of a remedy, I would be interested to know.

At the time when I came to this conclusion I decided that I could temporarily run away from it by occupying myself with hobbies, interests, travelling and work.

I would also brainwash myself by thinking that it was not important to have a child to carry on the family line. There was no guarantee that even if I had a child that we would be in each other's lives for whatever reason and that the continuity would necessarily be there. You see, as I said before, I will never take anything for granted again.

Would I want the worry and stress of raising a baby, having the energy to control a child, or being amicable towards them as adults? It is well-known that none of this is a piece of cake but as they say "I wanted to have my cake and eat it, too".

Eventually I woke up to the fact that I was not going be a mother. Final. There you are, I did it. My attitude would now be "what you don't know, you don't miss".

The most important thing now was for us to be focused and supportive of each other. Both Barry and I came to the conclusion that we wanted to be continuously healthy and happy, with many pursuits of current and new interests. We had our health. There were many people out there that did not. On the other hand there were many healthy people out there that had children. Do you get my gist? There was always that other little voice.

By Christmas we had come to the decision that we would pursue the fertility treatment one more time during the spring and then knock it on the head as I would be 42 on my next birthday in June. The finishing line was set in order to maintain our sanity.

Chapter Ten

Since the last miscarriage, like the sun rising in the morning on cue from the East, my period would each month arrive on its expected date. All my adult life, until the last seven years, that would please me. Maybe I was being punished for playing God, having used contraception over the years. Who knows? Daft thoughts like that often entered my mind.

I would have to face up to the fact that "the apple would just not fall off the tree".

I was busy dealing with clients at work one January morning when I received a phone call from the fertility clinic advising me that my name was now on the top of the list for a donated egg. A year and a half had passed since we invested our £100 and to be honest we had actually forgotten all about it. We could now have the option of taking a donated egg or two and, if so, to proceed immediately with Ovran 30 (The Pill) to manufacture a false cycle, to meet with the donors, and to start the nasal spray. We were now to be placed in a new ballgame and I replied that I had to communicate with Barry on the matter.

Barry and I talked and talked that evening. This would be a huge thing to undergo, especially for me. At four in the morning after a lot of thinking we decided to go for it! We had to, for the reason that this was, as we saw it, to be our last shot at the apple through fertility treatment. We had gone this far so now we had to increase our chances.

I rang the fertility clinic the following morning and made an appointment for all the usual checks and to collect the prescription that would be required.

I sat in the waiting room for my turn to be examined via the scan units. For the first time ever whilst I sat in the waiting room I glimpsed at a young couple who were totally beside themselves with grief. They were hurriedly collected by the nurse who comforted them with kind words and were ushered behind close doors, never to be seen again.

I suddenly thought "shit, get me out of here!" The whole experience of what I was doing dawned on me. The overwhelming atmosphere was that many others in that room felt very uncomfortable and emotional.

My turn arrived and I exchanged pleasantries with the friendly radiographer who I had not seen for a while. She confirmed that all was fine with my internals and that I would be seen by a nurse for a quick blood test and to collect the prescription and paraphernalia concerning what I was to undergo.

I was pleased to leave that building that day and gave out a huge sigh of relief knowing that I had now come to the decision that this was to be the last big effort and, unexpectedly, with a gift. A donated egg would be given to me from a younger woman than myself. Surely it would work this time!

I felt a tinge of excitement by the time I returned home and analysed what was to occur within the course of treatment. So much so, my concentration level was near zero. Focusing on selling hospitality packages and tickets was a no go area that day!

I was to start taking the Ovran and to start the nasal spray to switch off the hormones. I remember doing this and then curling up on the sofa with a huge mug of hot chocolate. It had just started to snow and I thought today was going to be a day off from work, fertility anxieties and hearing different opinions from friends and family. I went to my huge collection of DVDs and picked out one of the biggest epics to fulfil my mind. It worked.

Barry returned home harassed and stressed by the ongoing traffic from the office and bluntly said that he was pissed off! He then belatedly remembered that I had gone to the clinic for the routine check up. I replied and confirmed that all was in line for us to start the next course of treatment.

His anxieties filtered over to me that this was definitely going to be different from the previous attempts. I agreed and we ordered our Chinese takeaway with hardly more said on the subject. I had made the conscious decision that day I was going to let nature take its course. The less, said the better!

A week after swallowing the Ovran tablets at the same time each day, I received a call from the clinic informing me of details of the donor egg to be given. I was given a brief description of the weight, height, eyes & hair colouring of the donor without a name and address which at that time was totally forbidden. (The laws have since changed.)

A date had been set for the end of February when the egg transfer would take place. Both the donor and I would now have a false bleed at the same time in order to ovulate at the synchronised time for the implantation.

Barry and I did have to undergo the rigours of the fertility injections and I was still taking enough oral drugs to accommodate the hormones and the lining of my uterus.

Everything was on tow. I went back and forth to the clinic so that I could be monitored for my scans and blood tests. We were about a week away from transfer when I received a call from one of the nurses who informed me that my donor had bottled out and that they would call me with an immediate replacement.

Words would not come out of my mouth. Believe me that is a rare scenario. I asked her to repeat what she was nervously trying to advise me. She quickly followed up by saying that no harm would be done for me to continue taking the Ovran and to continue my sniffing of the nasal spray.

She guaranteed that the next donor on the list co-ordinating with my blood type would be put forward. A replacement would be found as quickly as possible. Apologies were given but it fell on deaf ears.

I hung up the phone. So acute was the disappointment I swore the biggest obscenities possible at my sorry looking teddy-bear in the corner of my office. I was in total disbelief and extremely angry but at the same time I knew it was a situation that I had to control and that I had to stay in control of my emotions. I hated that more than anything. The positive spirit had to prevail no matter what.

The lingering impression of hours and days would continue into an oblivion of hope that a replacement would be found. Indeed it was another three days before it was confirmed via the phone that a designated replacement had been located.

During this phone call I was told that I had to go through the whole rigour again as if we were starting from scratch. I was so disgruntled but I knew that my temper had to be kept in check, however painstakingly frustrating the whole situation was, knowing that there was no guarantee of the result we so wanted. Both I and my hormones were raging!

I hated myself for having to rely on someone who I had never met or knew. I vowed there and then that I would not allow this scenario to reoccur. If we were to volunteer to pioneer through another course of IVF in the future, (which at the time we thought highly unlikely) Barry and I decided that we would do so alone with no third party involved. The whole process was stressful enough without the added worry of 'will they turn up or not'.

Feeling totally disconsolate and looking like a pregnant duck, being bloated from the drugs I had taken I could not wait for this course of treatment to be over. I was ready to give it all up there and then.

The egg collection date had been arranged for the 30 April 2002. It was inconceivable that we had actually started the treatment for this course of IVF at the beginning of February. It did not bear thinking about what the consequences were of taking the drugs for a longer period of time. I was told this was nothing to worry about. All very well but when it is your own body on the line it is not so easy to digest. As always at this difficult time I had to continue to be positive in mind in order to achieve the ultimate result.

Maybe it was intuition but this course of treatment did fail miserably. Only four eggs were collected and two fertilised which were transferred into me. After the two week wait my period came on like clockwork. Mercifully I did not even have to go through a pregnancy test.

The impact of what had not happened affected us both rapidly, compounded by the feeling of vulnerability. We were devastated. We had lost our fight. We had to accept this was the final curtain. We both wept openly and whispered to each other as to how unfair this all had been. Why were we being put through this charade? Indeed, it was not a charade. In reality we now knew that this meant that we would never have children. Our line would come to a blunt end. In most of us it is deep-rooted consciously or unconsciously that we will have children leading to grand-children. We now had to accept that this would not be the case for us.

We spent the whole of the day expressing our frustrations and emotions and talked for endless hours about what we could do to change our outlook on life as a whole. We also knew that it would take time, if ever, to totally accept the heartache of being childless.

We had to put plans in motion to detach ourselves from the urge to be parents. We had to cut ourselves off from pursuing fertility treatment and just go with the flow. Sex would have to become pleasurable and not regimental as it had become. We had to line up the plus points against the minus points of not being parents. We would have to divert our attention and energies to new projects and interests.

I had to stop reading newspaper and magazine articles announcing solutions to deal with fertility problems. This was easier said than done. In our case, as we did not know what was causing our infertility, I did keep some newspaper cuttings of people experiencing similar circumstances in order that we could seek advice and find answers to our questions.

It was now time to divert our attentions and to find peace from the whole baby agenda. We now had to start a new chapter of our lives and to embark on a new journey of acceptance of the hand we had been given. We had to put it all into perspective as difficult as it was, and find a sense of peace of mind. No words can describe the pain you experience mentally unless you are unfortunate to have made a similar journey. The pain indeed was for both of us. I know that Barry suffered even having to console me at the time of miscarriage but also at the same time hiding the obvious devastation and torment that he endured quietly, as most men do.

At the time of the miscarriage it is very easy for the woman to be recognised as the sufferer but indeed both partners are prisoners to this pure misery and loss. I know that Barry heard me cry myself to sleep many times but never complained and always tried to console me, at the same time with a heavy heart of not knowing what to do or say and how to "make it better" for both of us.

I know this to be a very common occurrence with infertile couples and one must give applause and far more credit to the other partner. Men may not carry the babies and physically lose them or even openly shed tears but mentally it is a far bigger strain than many let on. They too see other fathers with their offspring and they too feel the jealously or the difficulty in being in the company of their compatriots - unable to participate in fatherhood matters. It is not easy baggage to carry.

Chapter Eleven

The first thing on my agenda was to get myself fit and healthy. It was vital as I had started to look so fat and drab. My skin and hair had become very dry. More than anything I constantly felt bloated, tired, tearful and moody. The hormones had been working overtime. I knew that I had taken far too many drugs over the years to no affect but punishing the parts of my body which were invisible to the naked eye.

The slate had to be wiped clean. No more pills, injections and therapies. As well as mentally, my perception of physical attitude had to change.

We booked many weekend breaks and pursuits. Our main holiday during the summer had been arranged. We started to connect up with friends. We were regular visitors to concert gigs, cinema showings; we even went to many productions at the theatre, sometimes during a weekday matinee.

I found visiting beauty parlours for massages and generally being pampered very therapeutic. This did wonders to boost my low morale at certain times when required.

Family and friends also suggested that we should get a dog to divert our minds from our loss of fertility. Often Barry and I would feel irritated by the suggestion but knew deep down that people were embarrassed and awkward about our inability to have a child so the next best thing to suggest was to have a dog. It was incredible how many people made the suggestion. It was not quite on our agenda at that time as we knew we wanted to do some travelling and take time-out from any commitments and to just sort our heads out!

It was a time of becoming numb to everyone and everything that would remind us of parenthood. Difficult as it was our mindset was changing. We knew that we had far more freedom and it was time to take advantage of that.

Eventually we did succumb the following year in the spring to getting a dog but this was another 10 months away. Barry had always wanted one since being a little boy "The Old English Sheepdog" or "Dulux Dog". We browsed through the doggie books to decide which would be the most compatible one.

Eventually Barry came to a compromise by choosing a Polish Lowland Sheepdog which is a smaller breed but related. This also became an adventure of its own with plenty of ups and downs.

It must be the sign of the times we were put on a wait-list for this particular breed of dog. Eventually, after a 10-month wait, we were lucky to be told that we could look at a four week old puppy based in Cardiff. The dog had been born on 22 February 2002. We went and fell in love with it and after being approved by the breeders and told that he was a pedigree dog we were told he could be ours. We were to return on his eighth week to collect him. We called him Monty.

Monty kept us more than busy and occupied. We went to dog training classes and I wore out many pairs of trainers. I had walked more than I had done for many years. Whilst walking we would often be stopped in the street, people gazing at his endearing beauty and unique characteristics, enquiring what breed he was. We were very proud of him and whilst we were on holiday that year the breeders looked after him in our absence. We returned to discover that he had won "best in show" for puppies at the local dog show. We were very proud of his achievement and loved him dearly! Apparently in true Monty style he did not want to participate in the show but once at the hall itself he posed willingly, showing off all his qualities and we were told he was a natural.

We thought about showing him for a while but we had acquired Monty as a pet and to nurture and love him in the safe haven of our home. We were determined to do this and to find other occupational hobbies that perhaps could also involve our dog.

It was during June that summer approaching my 42nd birthday that quite bizarrely I received a phone call out of the blue from the woman fertilitist/consultant who had helped us become pregnant on our first attempt at IVF. She was wondering how both Barry and I were coping as she had not heard anything from us. I told her that I thought we had knocked the whole fertility treatment process on the head. I mentioned that I had read an article that The Park Hospital in Nottingham had a successful pregnancy rate for older women and that Barry was originally born in Nottingham himself. She suggested that should we contact the Park Hospital she would gladly send a letter of referral should we require it.

On impulse I made an appointment for both Barry and I to visit The Park Hospital in Nottingham - also known as CARE at The Park. The appointment was made for Monday 8 July 2002.

The CARE Centres (Centres for Assisted Reproduction) are based at various hospitals throughout the UK. I had read that many of the consultants on the CARE team had been pioneers on all aspects of IVF - with many successes and achievements, including that of one consultant at CARE who was involved with the world's first IVF baby. Once at the hospital I was given a brochure and indeed inside were listed a mountain of firsts! I wanted my first! I was interested, very interested.

Whilst sitting in the very big bright sunny conservatory-like waiting room quite the opposite from what we had been used to in London, Barry and I looked at each other saying nothing. We knew somehow we were about to embark on a new journey. Would this be a happier and more positive one, were my desperate thoughts.

Once again we were expected to perform the usual basic tests. Barry had to embark on yet another sperm test and I had to undergo a couple of blood tests.

An appointment had been set with a specific consultant who could not meet us and instead we were introduced to another consultant who firstly apologised for whatever reason that the original consultant was not able to see us and then proceeded to go through our history of medical notes. He sympathetically listened to our queries, scepticism and anxieties. He concluded by giving us the option of talking to another consultant, George Ndukwe, who specialised in "inexplicable non-pregnancy cases and is in charge of the recurrent implantation failure clinic" and gave rave reviews of the achievements that had been ascertained from George's involvement, research and knowledge. "He is your man - please at least listen to his theories and have a chat with him."

The consultant excused himself from the room in order to see if it was possible for George to see us there and then.

He returned to us with a disappointed expression - unfortunately for us George was not available to see us that afternoon but he almost pleaded with us to make an appointment to see George after our return from our forthcoming summer holiday.

He concluded our meeting and confirmed that he would write to our doctors in London preparing them and us with the endless list of blood tests which had to be performed so that the medical operatives in Nottingham could investigate and break down the reasons of our infertility.

Before our next visit we also would have to undergo the screening tests that were required, namely HIV, Hepatitis B and Hepatitis C, together with our blood groups.

A couple of days later, after we had returned to London, I received a phone call from The Park Hospital confirming that an appointment had been set with George for the 30 September at 2.00pm.

At that time both Barry and I were really focused on our forthcoming holiday. We were treating ourselves to a really luxurious holiday in Northern Greece away from the hustle and bustle of everyday monotony and tedium. We had specifically saved up for the holiday after what we had undergone six months earlier and indeed over the previous six years. The highs and lows had hit us both hard.

We decided to put the whole of the Nottingham saga on the back boil. Little did we know it at the time, but on this particular holiday fate was about to show its hand once again.

Chapter Twelve

We had a lousy journey over to Greece that year and I remember that we were delayed. On our arrival at the hotel we were greeted and escorted around the hotel and I remember that we each received a glass of champagne (my inner thoughts were for just arriving in one piece) before we finally relaxed in our exquisite hotel room with a complimentary bowl of fruit and local delicacies.

For a couple of days the weather was beautiful but became extremely hot and humid even by Greek standards. After breakfast one morning the daylight became night and we made a dash back to our room before the heavens opened. The rain pelted down on our balcony and we stepped out like two nervous pigeons wondering what our next move was to be. It was very hot - about 95 degrees - even though it was raining hard amongst the backdrop of thunder and lightening.

Whilst out on our balcony we heard a family of English voices and leaned over the railings and started to join in with their conversation. The parents were about our age and they had a girl around 14 and a boy around 10. We started to chat in the rain whilst the kids were messing about with their gadget toys. Like us they were deciding whether or not to drive to the local town or take a chance on waiting for the skies to clear in the hope of catching the much needed rays of sunshine.

The decision was made that yes there was no point hanging around as the hotel did not have that many facilities to occupy us for the whole course of the day.

The family had a rented car and offered us a lift but we declined as it was a small car and we did not want to impose on them.

We went to the reception to order a cab but to our bitter disappointment there were no more cabs that would come out to the hotel for another hour or so due to the shortage of cabs available and hazardous conditions. A man overheard our plea and invited us to join him and his partner for a ride as they were going to a town nearby. It turned out that they were new Londoners originally from Iran and lived near us and we had a very interesting journey to the nearby village, both visually and vocally.

Once there we decided to meet at a set time for our return journey back to the hotel and started to walk off on our own only to discover that the shops were closed (not that there were many - and mainly tourist traps for knick-knacks). Disappointingly there was not too much to see and do. It was lunchtime so we decided to go to a local tavern which was open and situated on a beautiful spot overlooking a small harbour, albeit under canvas due to the heavy rain.

Coincidentally, the only family sat at the restaurant were the original family we had briefly spoken to earlier at the hotel on the balcony. They encouraged us to join them for lunch and we accepted the offer.

We introduced ourselves properly and it turned out that they were from Ascot. Once over the pleasantries and when we knew each other's names and what all our occupations were, where they were from and so forth, inevitably the question then to follow was "Do you have any children?" I then responded that we did not but we were considering a course of IVF treatment. They asked where. To which I responded "Nottingham". The response was amazing! "Our two kids were born through a course of IVF and it was at Nottingham - at the same clinic".

Both Barry and I were in total disbelief. They quickly followed up by saying "Do not hesitate - even if you have doubts - go with it, it will work!" Even the two children were enthusiastic and encouraged us to go ahead with Nottingham.

Over the years they had returned to Nottingham for a reunion get-together and could not praise the staff enough.

We devoured a good lunch even though we sat through a massive thunderstorm. We were probably there for a good two hours talking like long lost friends. We all came to the conclusion this was God's way of helping us make the decision to go ahead to pursue the new course of IVF treatment at Nottingham.

Even though they had undergone the treatment at a younger age they still insisted age did not come into it. They pointed out that if you want a baby this hospital will help you. They too had tried many hospital/clinics in the London area to no avail. We had nothing more to loose by listening to what the clinic would suggest for us. They felt very confident that even though we were clinically diagnosed "inexplicable" they would find a route problem.

As holiday friends do we spent a lot of time with each other, talking about previous experiences from life in general - hitting it off really well.

At the end of the holiday we exchanged phone numbers but unfortunately the bit of paper I wrote the number on became mislaid and they were X directory and we never heard from them. Individually they made me promise them that any doubts we had we should diminish them and to proceed whatever, and if I was to be successful I should let them know.

It was the end of August when we returned and the original appointment had been set for 30 September to meet George and both Barry and I felt far more positive about things even before we met him. Our friends in Greece had given us something very important. Hope and the much lacked positive thinking!

It was truly hectic on our return. We knew that time was of the essence and that we could not afford to let any more elapse to diminish our chances even more. No matter what, that appointment would be met.

Chapter Thirteen

We took a leisurely drive down the familiar M1 on a bright autumnal day. We decided to leave during the morning so that we could have lunch in the centre of Nottingham before making tracks to the clinic to meet Dr George Ndukwe, our consultant.

Once at the clinic, on time, we were shown into our consultant's room. We were greeted by George, a very tall and imposing man with a softly spoken voice. He immediately reassured us that for reasons which he explained, he was not prepared to put us through another session of IVF without first thoroughly investigating the reasons for our failures. He was endeavouring to prevent us from wasting further money and heartache, and both of us warmed to him immediately.

He further explained that he was in charge of an investigatory department that worked in close liaison with a Chicago hospital, headed by a well respected expert called Professor Alan Beer.

He felt confident that together they would pinpoint the reasons why conceiving and miscarriage were proving to be a problem for us.

He went on to explain that the most common reason for this was that the natural killer cells within the body could be attacking the embryo or placenta.

He also pointed out in order to fall pregnant and not to miscarry there are a course of five treatment categories but I may only need to follow one or two.

There would be 60 blood tests for me, the results of which would be sent over to the Clinical Immunology Laboratories at the Chicago Medical School, USA and which in close liaison with Nottingham would give results. From those findings the possible causes would then be taken on board, leading to the correct action to be taken in order to rectify the problem.

The added bonus in trying to trace the problems was that we had proof from the previous pregnancy loss. The remnants from the miscarriage could undergo tests and results produced from those findings.

This all sounded very encouraging to Barry and I and we knew that a new journey was about to commence to endeavour to find out "why"! This had never really been done previously in our quest to have a baby. It was just a case of you are not getting pregnant by yourselves so we will give you a treatment of IVF; even after failure we will give you more IVF - never mind the pocket and heartbreak for the poor couple involved. We were now in a different ballgame and truly a recommended one!

Appointments were made for the mountain of blood tests that had to be taken to pass on to Chicago. At a guess without going into the graphics it was not too dissimilar to having a transfusion. It was one long big blood test lasting for about 20 minutes. I teased the nurse that due to so many blood tests taken over the recent years that she may have to search for blood never mind trying to find a baby! Barry also had to undergo blood tests on a smaller scale.

I contacted the consultant who carried out the D&C operation from my first miscarriage. Thankfully the evidence was to hand from the loss we had suffered and this would further enable the laboratories in their quest for answers. This was a big plus! In the end all that to-ing and fro-ing with the D&C treatment proved to be invaluable.

The tests would take several weeks to be processed and evaluated. Once the results were available we were to be informed by Professor Alan Beer from Chicago by a three-way telephone consultation which would be set up by appointment. This call would be essential in order to discuss the significance of the test results and to outline the treatment plan in order to rectify the problems of pregnancy. Nothing prepared us for what was to come next!

After a couple of weeks had passed we received a telephone call from Alan Beer from the States. He introduced himself and was extremely friendly and had a relaxed style. I called Barry to pick up the receiver from another extension within our house so that he could listen and join in the conversation.

Looking back it was an original phone call in every aspect as both Barry and I had never been diagnosed by a specialist over the phone.

He started the phone call by confirming that we did indeed have to undergo the full five treatments. Picking up on both Barry's and my cursing he proceeded to say that this would not necessarily be a problem as he confidently felt that they now knew the route of all our problems and it would certainly be worth our while to pursue the treatments. Basically what it entailed was an extra intake of drugs to counteract the effect of the natural killer cells and to suppress the immune system within the uterus, at the same time protecting the foetus and placenta in its growth.

There were many reasons given for the added treatment, one of which stands out very fresh in my mind. One of the biggest reasons for the rejections was that the results from the tests concluded that incidentally both Barry's and my genealogy was so similar that it added to the barrier of conception. (HLA)-DQ Alpha Alleles. In simple language - if you are related it is far harder to produce a child. By the way for the record we were not related pre-marriage!

Alan Beer further informed us of his discoveries and expertise on immune evaluation and like a fortune teller commented on the medical history of our parents from the past and current without having met them. Astonishingly he was extremely accurate in his revelations.

Rheumatoid Arthritis was one of the symptoms diagnosed as being a main factor to my failure in becoming pregnant and indeed does run very strongly within my family genes. As I understand it, this is a proven factor for pregnancy loss or infertility.

The same applied to Barry who, as a teenager, had Crohn's Disease. Both of these symptoms alone are classified as Autoimmune Diseases which can produce blood-clotting disorders, a common contributory factor in pregnancy loss.

Alan Beer was so confident that he predicted I had a 70 – 90% chance of becoming pregnant which, compared to previous chances I had been given, seemed totally unbelievable.

He ended our conversation by confirming the approximate cost of the treatments to be carried out and that obviously the decision lay with us whether or not to proceed with the recommended treatment.

One of my personal concerns was the fact that this treatment was going to break my immune system down and that other illnesses and ailments would be free to filter through the body and I asked the direct and obvious question: would that also mean that there could be a chance that cancer cells can seep their way through the body?

He reassured me that from the tests taken there were currently no signs that this would happen and that my immune system would only be down temporarily. Viruses may possibly have more freedom to develop than previously but at the same time, and most importantly for us, the floodgates would be open to pregnancy.

I nervously asked the question was my age a problem. I was now aged 43. "Age does not come into it" was his reply. "Your immune system, as it is, does!"

Alan very confidently reiterated that our chances of becoming parents were as close to a definite as could be. He sympathetically answered all our questions of scepticism. Both Barry and I expressed our anxieties from the previous experiences we had already undergone. He was not at all surprised or fazed. He furthermore offered us the opportunity to call him at anytime in the future with any other questions we may have forgotten to ask or, if we decided to go ahead, to ask questions during the treatment itself.

He ended the conversation by wishing us luck with whatever we should decide and hoped that one day we would have the opportunity of meeting up.

The decision to be made now was ours. We knew from George that Alan had treated many women who had endured multiple IVF failures and numerous miscarriages, with a huge success rate, including women in their 40s. We knew this would be our last chance to create a family of our own. We knew from listening to this understanding and caring man that the decision would come to us easily. It was to be a green light or possibly better still, the beginning of the light at the end of a very long tunnel!

Chapter Fourteen

An appointment was made for me to undergo a Remicade Infusion which meant I would be a day-patient at the clinic in Nottingham. Prior to having Remicade I had to undergo a chest x-ray to rule out TB as the two are contraindicated. The use of Remicade is a costly treatment as it is not readily available in the UK. I was told that this would reduce the Rheumatoid Arthritis symptoms that I had incurred over the years and that I would feel better physically in the next couple of months. Almost super-human as said by someone - your joints and movement will be less stiff. Bring it on!

This particular treatment also fights the natural killer cells bringing down the immune system. The procedure entailed lying on a bed with an intravenous drip for about six hours.

We arrived at the clinic and were escorted to a private room where we were greeted by a very friendly nurse, originally from Wales. She handed me a gown to change into as the anaesthetist was to shortly insert the intravenous drip within the veins of my right arm.

I remember this nurse well. She was a positive person with an extrovert personality but at the same time not too over-bearing and left me with the peace and tranquillity of the room I was based in.

Barry went for walks in the nearby countryside and of course searched for that little pub to supply him with his fix!

The nurse loved her Rugby Union and excitedly told both Barry and I she was looking forward to seeing her team play a big match over the forthcoming weekend which we discussed at length amongst other things during the day.

She told me that many of the patients that had undergone this treatment did indeed fall pregnant, and the parents often brought in their offspring to show. She had a strong gut feeling that the same would apply to us. We promised that if we were successful we would be happy to do the same.

I was trying to stay positive but at the same time sceptical as I had been down a long road approaching my eighth year of various treatments.

I must admit it was a long boring day but generally painless other than the discomfort of the actual needle insertion and removal of the drip itself and having to endure the daytime soaps on the television or some magazines going over the latest diet, celebrity gossip or fertility or infertility suggestions!

From the infusion itself I had no side-effects to speak of. At the end of the day I was given a little alert card (not unlike a blood donor card) to put into my purse to advertise the fact that I had undergone a Remicade infusion so that should I be involved in an accident or to have an emergency operation for whatever reason, the medical staff concerned would be made aware.

We were now ready for the full IVF treatment that was to follow in a few weeks but this time with the help of the immune treatments.

I had started taking aspirin and calcium tablets. Injecting subcutaneously twice daily Clexane together with Prednisolone tablets, Folic Acid, vitamin B6 and Vitamin B12 for starters! All these would help reduce the risk of miscarriage after conception. The rattling inside my body was like a thunder drum. On the outside everything was crossed!

I do recall an amusing situation in taking all of these tablets and the down regulation (sniffing). It was already a cool dark November evening and as I was told to take things at a slower pace I remember after finishing some work at my desk, I made a brew and put my feet up in our lounge. I flicked through the TV channels and ended up watching "London Tonight" (a local London magazine programme). The announcer was speaking of an opportunity through a phone-in for a selected few to win the chance of meeting David Beckham at a private book signing of his biography "My Side". I don't know what made me do it but I did ring and left my details.

The following day I received a phone call from the television company to inform me that I had indeed won and that I should go to Waterstone's in Piccadilly. I was thrilled! I had never won anything before through a phone-in.

I remember that day like yesterday. It was a typical grey-skied rainy morning once I arrived in the West End. I decided to drop into Fortnum and Masons for an early lunch since I did not want the temptation of visiting every shop in the West End and walking my feet off! I also had to adhere to the times of taking the drugs so it was easy to sit, eat and take – so I thought!

After lunch I took the medication at the prescribed time at my table - paid the bill and went to the ladies toilet to freshen up before going on to the book shop a couple of doors down the road.

I locked the door to the toilet but to my horror it would not unlock. There was no one else around. After fiddling and trying physically to free the door I stood there for a moment or two smiling to myself thinking the situation rather funny. After the longest 10 minutes had passed no one else had come in and time was beginning to run out for my anticipated meeting with Mr Beckham.

I then again flicked around with the lock and as I eventually unlocked it and became free someone else walked in. I made her aware of what I had just experienced and exited quickly in order to make my appointment. I was never so pleased to leave Fortnum's as I was that day!

Once at Waterstones I was greeted by representatives from the shop who escorted me to join a queue of people. As a guess from memory it was about 500 or so people and mainly female.

Standing in the queue the surrounding people started to talk to each other, including me. I started talking to a couple of ladies who like myself had never won anything before in their lives and joked at the same time it was still not totally exclusive since the bottom line we were all still queuing! The scheduled time we were given to be at the shop was 3.30pm and it was now fast approaching 4.00pm and my accomplices were concerned about being in time to greet their children from school.

At 4.00pm after plenty of talking and meeting all types of people I glanced at my watch and knew that it was an essential time for me to take some of the oral medication, including enacting the sniffing procedure.

We were told that we could not break away from the queue but at the same time the personnel in the shop handed over to some people a paper cup filled with water. The people who had been omitted were beginning to get thoroughly pissed off and asked the staff to provide more as we were all equals. It was laughable then and is now.

Fortunately for me I had been given a cup albeit half full, just enough to take the pills, which I did rapidly. One of the ladies I had spoken to was watching and curiously asked me if I had a medical condition as I was taking so many. I responded by telling her that I was on fertility treatment and followed it up with the sniffing procedure. This then produced many questions from a few in the queue line. I explained to them the benefits of what I was taking. They also enquired as to how long I had been doing IVF. I told them snippets of my story. "You should write a book!" was the response.

Once at the top of the queue I met the man himself and must say he certainly has an angelic aura like no other sportsman I had met previously. Again I was laughing to myself. He looked like how I had imagined "Jesus" to have been.

To me David looked stunningly better close up than I had seen before from watching him play on TV or live.

He looked gorgeous. He wore a beautiful heavy leather dark brown jacket which accentuated his shoulder length sun-highlighted blond flowing locks with sparkling, endearing blue eyes and a golden tan. In the wings Brooklyn, his son, was playing around with security staff but at the same time was watching us all with what I am sure was such curiosity.

I had a photograph taken with David by one of the staff on hand who seemed to take an age to take the picture, during which I joked and charmingly David laughed at my comments and touched my arm in passing. I joke today that that might have been an important touch!

I thanked him and left the shop clutching onto the precious signed book. Whilst walking through the hustle and bustle of the busy London street of Piccadilly heading for Green Park tube station making my way home I remember on this dark rainy grim November evening being fully lit up from the spark I had just encountered. A smile would not leave my face. I had enjoyed that day. It was interesting and fun - eating a delicious lunch at Fortnum and Masons, even being locked in the loo - swallowing all my pills and potions in a queue and meeting interesting people. It was worth it!

Chapter Fifteen

I received a telephone call from Nottingham to say that five eggs were retrieved and fertilised. Two embryos were to be transferred tomorrow. The date was to be 5 November 2003.

We had to be back in Nottingham early in the morning. We packed an overnight bag for any emergency.

Barry hates driving on motorways so I volunteered the drive up the M1 leaving home at 4.00am. I remember that morning like it was yesterday.

I regularly drive up the M1 to visit my in-laws with my husband so I know the bumps and turns within the road quite well. However, that morning it was still dark with the added ingredient of pea soup fog. The journey was generally in silence other than the sound of voices on the radio accompanied by easy listening music which did send Barry to sleep albeit with me from time to time waking him informing him where we were, or to assist me if I could not see clearly what was in front due to the fog.

Once we arrived at the clinic in Nottingham we waited in an extremely quiet reception before being ushered to a room so that I could strip. I was totally relaxed with no anxieties to speak off. The whole atmosphere was serene and personable. Perhaps all my experiences of having gone through the motions before meant that I just slid into a 'switch off get on with it' mode.

Before the actual transfer of the eggs to my body we were shown their appearance and size on a televised screen and very methodically I lay on a bed for the insertion to take place.

At the time I did find it amusing that suddenly there were three or four other females outstretched on their wheelie beds like myself waiting their turn.

I remember after the transfer had taken place that I was pushed to lie by a wall and facing another wall with all cartoon characters blatantly staring. Instead of feeling despondent about the insensitivity of the characters being around in the very childless atmosphere, I indeed felt very at peace with myself, serene-like. Instead of feeling that I had been invaded by the loss of privacy of my inner-self I felt as if I had just undergone a relaxing rhythmic body massage being totally relaxed in body and, most importantly, in mind. I was struggling to keep my eyes open and focused on the mural in front. Eventually I did succumb to sleep. My face had a smug faint smile according to Barry. There again I could have been just really tired due to the fact that it was still very early in the morning and I had driven a couple of hours from London.

I was given the all-clear to return home after an hour or so after the transfer.

Looking back I must admit I felt the most confident I had ever felt before at this stage. Now after years of IVF failure and being completely in the dark, the findings from all the scientific data with the correct medication had increased my chances of success by a massive 80%. Without the treatment I would never become pregnant.

I must salute the staff at Nottingham; they were definitely number one for installing confidence. You only had to hear of the repeated high success rates and the kindness and care they bestowed. "Your age is not a problem! So what! You may have tried six times before but some people have tried double that amount and succeeded! You now know why you could hold on to the babies with our help; it will work you see!"

All those comments and voices stayed with me over the long two weeks I would have to endure before knowing the result. It definitely helped to keep me optimistic and not fall into pessimism, which is a very easy route to take.

Whoever reads this account, the biggest tip I can give you is find out via tests whether or not you suffer from a blood clotting disorder so that a blood-thinning treatment can be given.

Most important of all we were now fighting my immune system in order not to miscarry. We had learnt that this phenomenon would be the main reason for many pregnancies leading to miscarriage whatever the age of the prospective mother. Age was not the main deficiency. Hopefully, someone will benefit through this new area of medical science. Public awareness of this is very poor and should be broadened to a wider public domain. The prejudices of age does incense me and at the end of the day if someone is diagnosed with "unexplained infertility", make sure that your natural killer cell count is not too high, together with low blood clot identity and you are more than likely to conceive and less likely to miscarry. Sounds simple really yet I was never told this from the start of my long journey in pursuit of having a baby. The loss of finances together with the lost time could have been far more easily avoided, not forgetting the mass of heartbreak caused.

Obviously there are other diversions such as quality of the woman's eggs, fallopian tube blockages and so forth. I deeply sympathize with this and I would understand the frustration that meets these obstacles.

My point is, if the medical profession can help me sort out problems that are not physically visible than there must be hope for the inadequacies that are visible. Insist on having tests even if it means using a strand of your hair! The tests will show.

It is a lottery to find the right doctor as some can be totally dismissive or sceptical of certain treatments. My belief too is that some just have not done their own research and can be ignorant of certain corners of infertility. Some doctors' attitudes are very bad in that they treat women as if they are not intelligent enough to know anything. Do your research, which is so readily available today - fire the questions and expect answers. Do not fall into the trap of trying again with no real conclusion.

Chapter Sixteen

We were approaching the testing date and my positive attitude continued until the actual day of performing the pregnancy test whereby due to previous negative results, for a brief nervous moment, I thought I was as likely to become pregnant as a chance of me to flying out on a spaceship to meet up with the extra-terrestrials I mentioned at the beginning of this book, even though no blood stains had appeared.

Once again I took the applicator test in the serenity of my bathroom and gaped with total amazement - I was pregnant. Two years had passed without even a sign!

I was excited, of course, but I did also have one foot on the ground. I had been here before and amazingly twice before being pregnant pre-Christmas. Christmas again was on its way! No doubt with my head spent more down the toilet bowl than enjoying the festivities of Christmas.

Once again I made all the necessary antenatal plans and appointments and telephoned the clinic in Nottingham to confirm my good news to them.

An appointment had been set up for me to have a blood test and pregnancy scan and to see George just before Christmas. This we carried through and I can remember to this day how pleased everyone was and in fact George had a cold and I was too polite to say "watch it - I don't want one of those right now!" I knew that my immune system was now at a low and this thought pattern would continue throughout my pregnancy.

I was given a prescription of what I had to take throughout the pregnancy and I had to pass a copy of it to the hospital where I was to have the baby delivered in London. Unfortunately for us, once back in London, we had a problem trying to attain a particular medication. Panic began to set in as the following day was Christmas Eve. In my mind I was meditating KEEP CALM, DON'T GET STRESSED ... THIS IS NOT GOOD FOR THE BABY ... YOU WILL GET THE MEDICINE SOMEHOW ... BELIEVE ... BELIEVE. YOU KNOW EVERYTHING IS A BATTLE BEFORE SMOOTHING OUT ... BREATHE SLOWLY ... THINK POSITIVE THOUGHTS!

The only option we had thankfully was that the clinic in Nottingham could provide it and the only way forward was for the medication to be handed over to my mother/father-in-law. They lived in Nottingham. Luckily since they were spending Christmas with us, they were able to bring it with them to London.

I gave directions to my in-laws of where the clinic was located and they made their way there to be greeted by George at the reception area. He handed over the medication to my mother-in-law who in turn asked "will it work Dr George - my children have gone through so much already". He in turn replied "it is now in God's hands and in mine!"

Christmas came and went without any hitches and yes I was nauseous but luckily never physically sick. An appointment had been made for us to go back to Nottingham in the first week of January for a second early pregnancy scan which indeed re-confirmed that a baby was clearly visible. My due date was to be 12 August.

I was now eight weeks pregnant but I still had to fight through the medication to enable the baby to survive.

Under doctor's orders I continued to take a low dose of aspirin and to inject myself with Clexane, which I had been instructed to do throughout the pregnancy in order to fight the antibodies. This I did religiously daily - inserting the needle into my bits of flab, either on my hips or indeed even into my abdominal area or thighs throughout my pregnancy becoming more bruised as well as huge!

It became a race - I had to beat the antibodies to reach my first target of being pregnant longer than the 13 weeks that I had achieved previously. It was at this point that I had been prescribed to wean myself off the Prednisolone - so that by my 13th week I could stand on my own feet having reached a new pinnacle. This was a battle against the killer cells, the enemy who without these drugs would kill my baby.

I was also prescribed to continue to take Folic Acid, Vitamin B6 and B12.

Looking back to that time I now recall that I was reassured to a degree by taking the medication as prescribed, which instilled me with a new confidence and purpose.

More importantly than anything, Barry and I had sought to determine the reason why we had not been fortunate to have a baby.

We had now been given some answers. My immune system had to be broken. The medication was the aid to help us fight against the antibodies which had always attacked my pregnancies. I also grew in confidence as I had not undergone most of the instructions/ medication throughout any of my previous attempts. It was new optimism. My race could now be won. I had a true chance.

From now on I was to be scanned, monitored and treated in London just like any regular pregnancy. Our financial resources had truly been evaporated from the endless IVF treatments we had undergone so we continued to receive treatment on the national health scheme.

My first appointment would be a month later on 2 February - 12 weeks into the pregnancy.

Barry accompanied me on this visit and we checked in all my details and medical history to the Antenatal Clinic at St. Mary's Hospital, in London. I informed them of the medication I was prescribed and they in turn welcomed me to participate in antenatal classes, nutrition benefits and other relevant topics.

We were introduced to a doctor and after a considerable wait I briefed him on the full history of previous pregnancies and to be aware of the treatment I was currently undergoing and suggested that if they were not sure of this latest IVF treatment, to contact Nottingham.

As I was categorised as an older mother the doctor felt sure that I would have a Caesarean section (C-Section) to waive any insecurity I gave out with regard to giving birth. I did not really pay much attention to finding out about other ways of giving birth.

Those early child-like memories still echoed my fear of childbirth which was beginning to come to the forefront but deep down I was still fighting those demons. My main focus was to be pregnant and to hold on to it. I would deal with the delivery of the baby and cross that bridge when came to it, should I be lucky to do so.

I was told that the choice was mine with regard to giving birth naturally or to have the C-Section. Being inexperienced in this area I was unsure and confirmed that I would inform the hospital as soon as I had made the decision. Although at the later stages I was to discover this did not apply at all.

The doctor also reassured us by suggesting that if I or Barry had any questions or anxieties to contact any of midwives/doctors within the hospital day or night. The doctor confirmed that my pregnancy now would be treated like any other pregnancy but all the IVF details had been noted.

The scan then followed and to my amazement the foetus had grown on the pictures quite substantially since the last scan I had viewed in Nottingham. The scan revealed a good sized baby with a strong and regular heartbeat. Just in four weeks I could now see a baby, my baby! We were asked if we would like to know the sex of the baby. We turned down the offer and concluded we liked the element of surprise. It was then that my excitement became almost unbearable.

Following the scan I also then had a couple of blood tests/urine samples which were to be analysed for Downs Syndrome. We were also booked in for a further scan and blood tests and my pregnancy would be monitored on a monthly basis. We were recommended by a very friendly receptionist to make our appointments there and then, due to the high volume of mums-to-be!

I reached my pinnacle of thirteen weeks with no problems and a week or so later received confirmation that no Downs Syndrome risk had been detected.

Thankfully, after the rigorous treatment of IVF I had undergone, the pregnancy blood tests and scans from therein would be a doddle.

At last I felt healthily pregnant and celebrated by embracing the baby departments within the shops. I was now, after all those years, looking out for prams and baby furniture. I had joined the baby wagon!!

The only difficulty I had over the coming months was parking outside the hospital.

There were endless amounts of traffic wardens parading the streets of Paddington; more than I had known anywhere in London. The traffic wardens would zoom in like vultures on any car a second over its time-limit. A prime target for them would be out-patients who would have to sit minutes or even hours longer than their arranged appointment times thus the ticket warden would be in good business.

I remember several times whilst trying to get a meter watching endless disagreements and fights with traffic wardens outside the hospital.

One comes to mind when a very normal looking 30ish man came out of the hospital accompanying his very heavily pregnant lady. Her face was distinctly grimacing with discomfort. The man had his arm around her left shoulder ushering her into their car. The warden was writing out his ticket rapidly, totally ignoring the existence of the couple. He showed no courtesy or acknowledgement of the fact that it was an emergency get-away. The warden was standing in front of the main window-screen lifting up the wipers to insert the hurriedly written ticket. The man then emerged angrily from the car. They had a few verbals and the man out of the blue smacked the warden, who landed on his bum pathetically, on the edge of the kerb.

I would normally have felt some sympathy for the warden but not in this case, as I had seen too many similar scenes and incidents outside this particular hospital over the months. I whooped and hollered and once the man had left that particular space I now had the vacant parking space after a long, but fully entertained wait.

Another memory from my scan visits to the hospital was a first-hand viewing of two uniformed prison guards accompanied by a very heavily pregnant loud-mouth cockney-spoken burley woman in her 30s with a shimmering set of handcuffs binding her wrists. She was sitting in the waiting room waiting for her turn to have a scan and informing every nurse that she was going to find out the baby's sex and said "I hope that it will be a boy this time". Her turn came and when she emerged from the scan she broadly announced to all of us - "it's a bloody girl again, my old man is going to kill me as he wanted a footballer!" Barry burst out laughing, finding the situation amusing. All I could keep thinking about was how easy it is for people to take for granted having a baby, and only be concerned about what sex it would be. Never mind the fact that she was extremely lucky to have any and that so many good people, for whatever reason, could not. The prisoner was then ushered out by the wardens and security staff - never to be seen or heard again!

The rest of my pregnancy was quite uneventful. I was monitored all along through phone calls and regular monthly checks to the antenatal clinic.

I continued taking the aspirin and vitamins and admit I felt very good throughout most of my pregnancy, barring one weekend retreat to a hotel just outside of London. It was during a May bank holiday weekend and I was in my seventh month of pregnancy.

The hotel was beautiful and excitedly we arrived on the Saturday lunchtime for a spot of lunch and a walk around the hotel's golf course. We retreated to our bedroom for a nap, which we did not succeed in having as the beds turned out to be very hard. A definite 'no no', as it was extremely uncomfortable if you were pregnant. We decided to watch a bit of TV and to Barry's delight a good football match was showing.

We had made a dinner reservation in the hotel's renowned gourmet restaurant and ate the most delicious meal. After returning to our room the quest was on for me to get comfortable on the bed to have a good night's sleep. After tossing and turning for a couple of hours, I whispered to a sleepy husband that I was going to take the car and drive home for what was left of the night for some kip. Baby and I desperately needed the sleep. We lived no more than 30 minutes away. It worked!

I returned refreshed the following morning in time for breakfast. It was a beautifully laid out buffet with plenty of choice. I ate a hearty breakfast but didn't overdo it! It was not long after finishing that Barry and I checked out and made our way home. On the journey back I felt very nauseous.

We literally just walked in the front door with me running to our toilet for a never-ending vomiting session. This continued throughout the day. My worry was that I was becoming dehydrated and of course was worried about the health of the baby.

I called a doctor at the hospital. The doctor's analysis over the phone (as it was Sunday) was that I had contracted violent food poisoning. He diagnosed that I should stay put in bed for the rest of the day and to keep taking plenty of liquids. At the time it was pretty scary but I did live to tell the story!

So much so the following day through a telephone conversation with my mother I had learnt that another couple of a friend of my mother's had also contracted food poisoning at the same hotel over the weekend. Both she and I later found out that we had both eaten some dodgy lamb.

Chapter Seventeen

The rest of May and June passed without any further incidents. Thankfully the weather during those months was bearable. It was not uncomfortably hot.

We went for our final scan and we were given the option of knowing the sex of our unborn baby. I had a very vivid memory of the prisoner that had been escorted into this room a few months earlier.

We were greeted by an oriental radiologist who led us to a dark dingy little corner room. She was softly spoken and busily writing down notes. She silently scanned my tummy, and I could clearly see the most welcoming picture on screen. The room to me now became very bright. Barry excused himself to go to the bathroom. In his absence the radiologist lifted her head away from her written notes. She enquired if we would like to know the sex of the baby. I responded by suggesting we wait until my husband returned before making a decision. I was mesmerised by what I was seeing on the monitor and scrutinising to see what I could on the screen with baited breath. The excitement was too much to bear. This time we succumbed and to our delight were told that it was a girl.

I could not believe it as I was convinced I was to have a boy. These were for total silly reasons. I was not too big out at front. I had decided on a boy's name. I had a selection of girl's names.

Also on this visit at the beginning of July we were informed that the baby's position was not as it should be. It had not turned. We were reassured that this was nothing to be worried about and that it should flip over. An additional scan was arranged for the following week to see if there had been any movement.

We returned the following week for the promised scan with the additional appointment arranged to speak to a doctor. As it turned out the baby had not moved and the doctor explained that the danger was that the umbilical cord could hang out the reverse way to what it should. This would not be a good idea should I go into labour, and therefore they recommended that I be admitted to hospital immediately with the prospect of undergoing an emergency caesarean at an appointed time.

It was then that I found out that I was to undergo a normal delivery before all this had occurred. I had just assumed a caesarean delivery was on the agenda due to my age factor as previously mentioned by the other doctor on our first visit. I was wrongly led.

It was now very hot outside and I asked if I could be admitted after the weekend due to the heat and with my promise of not moving anywhere. I would be far more comfortable in my own bed as opposed to the hospital's. The doctor had already indicated the operation would not happen so quickly.

It also gave me the chance to pack my overnight bag with the goodies I would require for my stay at the hospital.

It was a Friday and on our way back home I felt a little apprehensive but at the same time pleased that I could sort things out for our early arrival. I did not have any discomfort other than feeling hot and had the most chronic craving for sour lemon ice lollies. Monty, our dog, would be on the receiving end of any droplets. He loved it too.

It was over two weeks before the expected due date. Barry and I discussed over the weekend names and eventually after much deliberation decided to pin it on one of three choices. We still had a little time to go.

It was over two weeks before the expected due date of 12 August. My admission date on Monday 27 July was a beautiful day, so much so that Barry took some video shots of me in the garden looking very pregnant.

I remember asking Barry if he was bringing the camera into the delivery room for pictures. I told him that I had no problem with that and he in turn responded by saying that he would in no way be filming the main event.

Admission into the hospital seemed to take an age, so much so I was in two minds to go straight back home as my tummy was tied in knots with nerves. Once in the ward Barry was ushered away and blood tests were given. The named wrist tag was tied on.

There were six beds in the ward - all curtains were drawn. Were there any people around? Suddenly my curiosity was answered. The screams of labour were hollowing all around. I was living my nightmare from my youth. I huddled into my 10ft by 8ft space and drew the curtains around me petrified! I sat on my bed and slowly undressed into my nightdress and unpacked some of my belongings onto a spartan side table. Above there was a television monitor and telephone console system which was hugely costly but a must for distraction. Mobile phones were forbidden but as I found out, the odd sneaky call could be made.

I started to read a magazine when a young doctor introduced himself and reassured me that everything was on track. I was to have a C-section delivery on Wednesday just two days away. I could not wait and thought how lucky I was since I was surrounded by the pain and misery of the onslaught of natural childbirth. With gritted teeth I prayed I would not go into labour!

The following day the weather outside had become very hot and inside the hospital it was very uncomfortable. Thankfully I had bought in some liquids, fruit and titbits to nibble but the food the hospital offered was only suitable for mid-winter's supper, being tasteless, very much like airplane food.

I had never slept on beds that were as hard. The mattress had a plastic covering under the sheet which made it extremely sticky and damp. The nurse reprimanded me harshly when I once tried to remove it. I had caused the sin of trying to make things comfortable and hygienic for the patient.

As for the showers and lavatories, I had never experienced anywhere let alone a hospital. Hygiene just was non-existent. The floor was strewn with toilet paper and urine puddles. Even on the odd occasion I was greeted to excrement stains being on the floor and smeared on the walls within the shower cubicle.

As well as having a baby and keeping cool physically and mentally, most important of all I had to prevent myself from acquiring the e-coli disease. My immune system had been broken in order to become pregnant in the first place. I was a prime target for viruses!

Sleep was also non-existent for me for so many reasons. It was hot and sticky, I was hungry and thirsty, the hard sweaty uncomfortable beds, the groans from adjoining patients. I also had my craving for the lemon ice lollies, which of course were nowhere to be had.

The biggest reason was the anticipation and excitement of the impending birth - my baby would be born imminently.

On Tuesday night or should I say Wednesday morning at 12.20 am my harassed doctor visited me and informed me that I would not be having the C-section as planned for Wednesday. I was to be informed later in the day of what the new time would be. It was then that I found out that I was never scheduled in for a C-section from my antenatal visits. I had been down as a patient going on the natural route, since my pregnancy had gone well.

The doctor informed me that I was a late C-section booking entry only from the discoveries of the previous week.

I thanked him for seeing me at such a late hour and thought to myself I was to be one of the lucky ones in having a C-section. When they are ready I will be more than ready I thought. I only had to hear the groans which I was surrounded with. My heart went out to those women!

On the Wednesday I befriended some of the other patients and we talked about anything and everything, including the surroundings we had to endure. We shared cooling fans which had been bought into the hospital from our loving partners. We would huddle in front of the welcomed air and took the opportunity to talk to each other.

Visiting times for relatives and friends were very limited, so it was truly a pleasure when anyone managed to slip in.

On one occasion I fell on my knees with sheer gratitude when my mother came in with a couple of boxes of lemon ice lollies to feed my current addiction. I also ended up sharing these with my fellow patients who were just grateful for anything refreshing and cool.

Finally after waiting much of that day it was confirmed that my delivery was to be the following morning at 9.00am. I asked if my mum could be there as it would be a long awaited day for her as much as for me.

Chapter Eighteen

After yet again a very long, noisy and hot night the morning could not have come quick enough. The sun was shining outside as much as I was inside, albeit tired but exhilarated.

It had been confirmed that I would be moved to the delivery side room at 9.00am. Barry and my mum arrived promptly at 8.30 accompanied by the camcorder that Barry had vouched no way he was using but it was there should it be needed. Whatever that meant?!

Just after 9.00 the attendees wheeled me out on my bed to a recovery room which was a pleasant enough room. Better than anything I had encountered on the three previous days of my stay. Nerves were beginning to set in as we were kept waiting for about an hour before a nurse gave Barry his gowns in order to watch the proceedings in the delivery room. Mum, being the maid-in-waiting, continued to stay in the room awaiting news of the impending birth.

Barry introduced his camcorder and asked permission if it could be part of the forthcoming operation. The staff had no qualms with this and added that it was now part of the proceedings.

Suddenly without knowing it my jaws did not stop moving. I was talking to anyone within eyesight. This is always the case when I am nervous.

Once we were in the operating theatre both Barry and I were introduced to the anaesthsist and surgeons who were accompanied by a couple of nurses. The obstetrician that had originally been scheduled to carry out the operation was unavailable. However, nothing could upset me that day and the information went straight over my head.

The procedure was quickly explained and before I knew it I was staring at a 12" long needle which dangled right before my eyes. I was told that this was to be the spinal injection which would numb me from the waist down.

The medical staff were bantering along merrily about their evening out the night before and conversing about cars.

The amusing part of the conversation turned to when they asked Barry whether or not we knew of the sex of the baby to be. Barry replied that we did and the obstetrician quickly responded "Don't tell me as I like surprises!"

They were also teasing Barry, who now had started filming the special event taking place. We still have the footage where I am sitting on the edge of the bed talking quicker and quicker whilst the disappearance of the spinal needle into my back is clearly seen. I am also holding on to the staff with clenched fists for support.

I was then told to lie down and to relax. This I did in a trance staring at the fluorescents above me, trying to comprehend all the conversation around me. I wanted to be relaxed and to remember every minute. I had waited for this moment for a very long time. In no way did I want to forget it and I was very grateful for Barry and the camera being there so that we could relive it in the future and for our child.

After a few minutes the surgeon touched parts of my body to see if I could feel anything. I was numb; however, I do remember once the operation had commenced feeling very light butterfly touches. Thankfully there was no pain.

All I could see was a board sectioned in front of me which had been placed so that I could not actually see the surgeons at work. I could also see the medical staff in their blues around the theatre. The anaesthetist was placed behind my head with his hands on my shoulder in conversation with Barry. Barry was unexpectedly also excitedly incessantly filming every minute.

I glanced towards the right of me and noticed a clock. It was 11.25. A couple of minutes later I heard a baby cry.

"IT IS INDEED A GIRL", were the words I next heard. Congratulations were given all around. There were plenty of handshakes and Barry stopped filming to kiss me and our newborn. No words can describe that moment. It was as if the whole world stopped moving. We were as in the movies "freeze frame" but truly very real.

A nurse asked me if we had chosen a name and if I wanted her tested for something (PKU) which I cannot remember as I was on another planet. I entrusted her to do whatever she had to and responded by shouting out to everyone. Her name will be Lauren. Lauren Rachel.

The nurse then went over to Barry and asked if he had a baby grow with him in order that the nurse could wash and dress the baby so that I could then hold her.

Meanwhile with all the emotions and activity around me the board was still up to separate me from seeing what the surgeons were doing. The two of them had gone very quiet and were busily trying to stitch me back.

At the end of the procedure the obstetrician was angry that he had not been informed via my notes that I had a huge amount of fibroids which had given them concern whilst pulling Lauren out. At the same time this had meant I had lost more blood than I should have, due to the length of time that had been taken for the procedure.

Finally, after being stitched up my darling Lauren had been returned to be held and she held my little finger with a strong grip trying to focus on me. She stopped crying. She was a true beauty. Well worth the wait. She had dark brown hair with long eyelashes. She weighed seven pounds.

Everyone asks if I cried. No, because I was in a bubble of disbelief. All I could do was stare at Lauren with a newborn curiosity, as much as she did towards me.

Barry returned to the theatre, which I did not even notice he had left to tell my mum of the news, who in turn relayed the news to my brother and his family.

Barry also telephoned my in-laws in Nottingham. Unfortunately for them my father-in-law had contracted shingles and at that time could not be present. Barry called them and said "We have got one!" They in turn replied not knowing that we had always known the sex of the baby asked "What have you got?" Barry excitedly shouted out "A girl, what I always wanted!"

Barry and I were totally mesmerised with the beauty of our baby. We concluded that the name we had chosen was definitely right and happily re-confirmed it for the registry.

I was wheeled back to the recovery room and was greeted by my beaming mum. She smothered me with kisses and expressed words of congratulations. She excitedly requested to see and hold her granddaughter for the first time.

My father was terminally ill at the time and very much in our thoughts. This was a very special moment for my mother. A relief for her from all the unhappiness she was enduring at home. Indeed it was a special time for all of us. The year had been especially difficult.

Whilst still in the recovery room I fell asleep. I was awoken by the sounds of the familiar voices of my brother and his family who on their visit were introduced proudly to the new member of our family. Lots of excitement filled the air and many pictures and cooing indeed took place.

Shortly after their visit I was ready to be returned to the maternity ward with my new addition.

Disappointingly, I was moved out of the original ward to a new ward with none of the familiar faces I had befriended during my previous week's stay.

A nurse came by and showed me the ropes with regard to breastfeeding and nappy changes.

Later on during the evening one by one each of the half dozen beds available became utilised.

I remember an Arabic lady coming in with an entourage and insisted on the windows being closed as she felt cold. It was 80+ degrees outside! Her entourage also closed the door to the entrance of the ward making it boiling! I also became over boiled with anger as after opening the door it was closed again. I decided to confront a nurse for some sort of compromise to be made for the sake of my baby and the surrounding others. I knew that overheating at the best of times could be dangerous and certainly during that night as it wasn't cold.

The hygiene as mentioned before was pretty much non-existent and with the heat it was most uncomfortable. I was praying for my release date to be sooner rather than later.

For the best comfort I stared proudly and endlessly at my beautiful baby girl. Lauren was sound asleep for most of the time.

She slept through all the commotion within the wards. The cries of labour and newborns hardly stirred her at all.

At about 2.30am an elderly maternity nurse looked in to see how we were doing. She volunteered to bring in a triangular pillow which she insisted would be an aid for my endeavours with breastfeeding. "Far more comfortable for you and baby" she would repeatedly say.

She kindly returned with the huge endearing pillow and performed a demonstration as to its usage.

About an hour later I suddenly had the urge to expel all the urine which I had held onto in order to prevent as many little visits to the inhospitable toilets.

Since it was the middle of the night and security was in place I took it upon myself to quickly leave the ward for the unwelcome visit.

I crept down the dimly lit corridor to the awaiting toilets. Opposite two nurses were sitting at a desk with a spotlight on. Once I had finished I went to the desk for a friendly chat to the two nurses on night duty. They started to talk to me when suddenly without warning everything started to spin round and one of them shouted out "catch her!" I apparently then passed out.

Following that incident I had been diagnosed as being anaemic, which was probably connected to the fact that I had lost more blood than normal. I now knew why the surgeon had been cross at the birth with the knowledge that no one had informed him of the impending masses of fibroids that had blocked the passage for Lauren's arrival which had led to the heavier loss of blood.

The following morning the doctor offered me the option of a blood transfusion or take oral medication to correct my blood count.

The decision was easy. I chose very quickly the latter option due to having witnessed the unpleasant surroundings and mistrust of the cleanliness within the hospital for the needles to be spotless!

MRSA was very much in the news and I knew that my immune system was low due to the conception treatment. The last thing I needed was to be a target for the nastiest of viruses.

The only downfall to having to take the oral medication was that a blood transfusion was a quicker remedy but I was no way taking the risk. My way of thinking was 'let's face it, I had been an expert for the last nine years in taking oral medication so what was another!' I now had a beautiful baby to look after and I wanted to be alive and well.

I had to stay in that wretched hospital for a few extra days due to the latest setback, which I had no option but to agree to.

I saw my colleagues within the hospital which I had befriended before delivery. We were each exchanging comments on the novelty of our babies and the experiences of what we had undergone for our welcome deliveries.

We were even more emotional than we were before the births, for obvious reasons and were truly exasperated with being in the hospital. Once we knew of our turn for departure from the hospital we would exchange telephone numbers. Sadly we never kept in touch.

Once the stitches had been removed from the C-Section and I had been given the all clear, my exit was very welcomed and swift.

Barry came to collect me and Lauren. Excitedly Barry once again produced the camcorder and filmed me and Lauren leaving the hospital which had been my home for 10 days and more importantly where we first set eyes on our lovely daughter.

Once outside it was raining. We did not have a care in the world. We were leaving the hospital with our baby which we never thought we were going to have. This experience was one which we both thought we would never encounter and here we were filming on the hospital steps with such pride our new bundle of joy!

Barry suddenly remembered through the excitement that our car, which was parked on a meter, had only a few minutes left to run. Desperately we did not want to incur any parking tickets on today of all days.

With our baby in hand we hurried through the streets of Paddington on a warm dark rainy August afternoon to prevent getting a parking ticket and not to be caught by the resilient traffic warden as I had witnessed so many times previous.

We beat the traffic warden and we beat the odds of our having the baby that we and so many people had given up hope on. It may have been raining that afternoon but as far as we were concerned the sun was truly shining on us.

Once home in our living room we introduced our new addition to our darling dog Monty who was just so glad to see me after the void of me not being at home over an eternity for him. He kept looking at Lauren with great curiosity and tenderness. He sat next to her baby carrier with an air of protection.

I felt at this moment that I had won the lottery; I was surrounded by my closest and dearest. To top it and most importantly of all Lauren had been born healthily. Unexpectedly she was born on 30 July 2004 not during the second week of August as first predicted.

I am very much a fatalist and this date, as I later discovered, was the same day those 38 years earlier the England football team had won the world cup as true winners of the world. With ecstasy of sheer joy and total disbelief we now had our trophy - the best in the world!

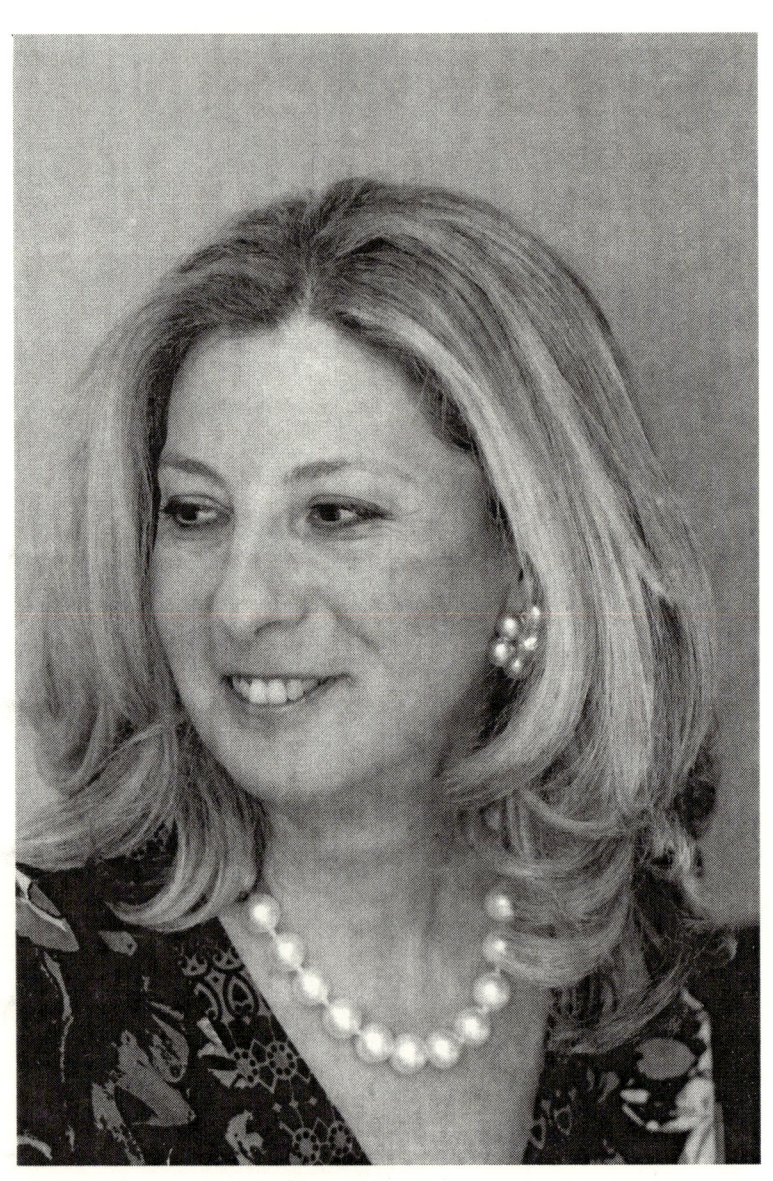

About the Author

Born in London Nicole Klieff is a first time writer. She was encouraged to put pen to paper by being inspired by her own personal experience of having undergone IVF treatment in a bid for a much longed baby. Due to the lack of information being readily available with a personal viewpoint she decided to write her own emotional story.

Acknowledgments

I should like to express my thanks to all those who helped me at CARE in Nottingham, with a huge thank you to the late Alan Beer and to George Ndukwe who made everything possible.

I would also like to thank everyone at Authorhouse for making this whole process an absolute delight.

*F*inally, for my husband Barry - just because. Thank you.

Printed in the United Kingdom by
Lightning Source UK Ltd., Milton Keynes
136740UK00001BA/4/P